CAMBRIDGE LIBRARY COLLECTION

Books of enduring scholarly value

History of Medicine

It is sobering to realise that as recently as the year in which On the Origin of Species was published, learned opinion was that diseases such as typhus and cholera were spread by a 'miasma', and suggestions that doctors should wash their hands before examining patients were greeted with mockery by the profession. The Cambridge Library Collection reissues milestone publications in the history of Western medicine as well as studies of other medical traditions. Its coverage ranges from Galen on anatomical procedures to Florence Nightingale's common-sense advice to nurses, and includes early research into genetics and mental health, colonial reports on tropical diseases, documents on public health and military medicine, and publications on spa culture and medicinal plants.

Biographical Memoirs of Medicine in Great Britain

In this absorbing work of medical history, the physician and writer John Aikin (1747–1822) brings together biographical information on a selection of Britain's early medics, shedding light on the lives, works and quirks of more than fifty medical writers, surgeons and physicians between the thirteenth and seventeenth centuries. Outlining the roles played by major figures in the great medical advances that marked this period, the book was first published in 1780, prior to Aikin's move to Great Yarmouth in 1784 to practise medicine. However, his political beliefs and dissenting views regarding the Church of England contributed to his unpopularity in the area, prompting his move to London and greater literary freedom. Over the years, he produced a broad range of published works, including his historically valuable *Description of the Country from Thirty to Forty Miles Round Manchester* (1795), which is also reissued in the Cambridge Library Collection.

Cambridge University Press has long been a pioneer in the reissuing of out-of-print titles from its own backlist, producing digital reprints of books that are still sought after by scholars and students but could not be reprinted economically using traditional technology. The Cambridge Library Collection extends this activity to a wider range of books which are still of importance to researchers and professionals, either for the source material they contain, or as landmarks in the history of their academic discipline.

Drawing from the world-renowned collections in the Cambridge University Library and other partner libraries, and guided by the advice of experts in each subject area, Cambridge University Press is using state-of-the-art scanning machines in its own Printing House to capture the content of each book selected for inclusion. The files are processed to give a consistently clear, crisp image, and the books finished to the high quality standard for which the Press is recognised around the world. The latest print-on-demand technology ensures that the books will remain available indefinitely, and that orders for single or multiple copies can quickly be supplied.

The Cambridge Library Collection brings back to life books of enduring scholarly value (including out-of-copyright works originally issued by other publishers) across a wide range of disciplines in the humanities and social sciences and in science and technology.

Biographical Memoirs of Medicine in Great Britain

From the Revival of Literature to the Time of Harvey

JOHN AIKIN

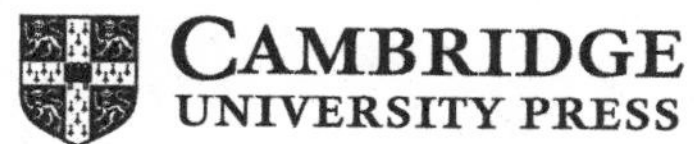

CAMBRIDGE UNIVERSITY PRESS

CAMBRIDGE
UNIVERSITY PRESS

University Printing House, Cambridge, CB2 8BS, United Kingdom

Cambridge University Press is part of the University of Cambridge.
It furthers the University's mission by disseminating knowledge in the pursuit of education, learning and research at the highest international levels of excellence.

www.cambridge.org
Information on this title: www.cambridge.org/9781108075947

This edition first published 1780
This digitally printed version 2015

ISBN 978-1-108-07594-7 Paperback

BIOGRAPHICAL MEMOIRS

OF

MEDICINE

IN

GREAT BRITAIN

FROM THE REVIVAL OF LITERATURE

TO THE TIME OF HARVEY.

BY JOHN AIKIN, SURGEON.

---- Genus innocuum, vitæque ad publica nati
Commoda, divinas tantúm didicere per artes
Exercere ævum, atque humanæ præesse saluti.

FRACAST.

LONDON:

PRINTED FOR JOSEPH JOHNSON, N°. 72, ST. PAUL'S CHURCH-YARD.

MDCCLXXX.

PREFACE.

THE Volume here preſented to the public is not ſuch as the author wiſhed it, but ſuch as he has been able to make it. Inſtead of a complete *Medical Biography of Great Britain*, he has been obliged to confine himſelf to ſome *Biographical Memoirs of Medicine*; and theſe, inſtead of deriving from obſcure and antient records, he has drawn only from ſources opened *ſince the revival of literature.* How far his plan is really the worſe for this deviation, he ſubmits to the judgment of each reader; but he thinks

 himſelf

himſelf obliged to ſay a few words reſpecting the *cauſe* of it.

THE firſt circumſtance which made him ſenſible of having ſketched out a plan beyond his abilities fully to execute, was the peruſal of Dr. Milward's *Invitatory Letter*, publiſhed in 1740; the deſign of which was to ſolicit the aid of the learned in compoſing juſt ſuch a work as that projected by himſelf. The numerous and abſtruſe objects of enquiry ſtarted in this pamphlet, are ſufficient to deter any perſon from the purſuit, who is not poſſeſſed of a great deal of knowledge and leiſure, together with the opportunity of free acceſs to every help for ſtudying ſucceſsfully queſtions of remote antiquity. Accordingly, it appears from the event, that Dr. Milward's ſcheme was unfiniſhed and forgotten.

THE aſſiſtances the preſent writer had flattered himſelf with the hope of obtaining,

obtaining, by means of his *Addreſs to the Public*, fell ſo much ſhort of his expectations, that even had the ſubject been much leſs extenſive, he muſt have abandoned the proſecution of his original deſign. He ſoon perceived, that of all the materials for information, *printed books* were alone what he had any chance of procuring. This, at once, reduced his plan to the compaſs of a comparatively modern period. He was further mortified with the proſpect of not accompliſhing even *this* part of his deſign ſo perfectly as he thought to have done. After the moſt extenſive enquiries, many of the publications he had liſts of were no where to be found; and a few, though known to exiſt, were locked up in libraries, the rules of which did not allow of their being lent for peruſal, on any intereſt or ſecurity whatſoever.

AFTER this free confeſſion, it will probably be aſked, "Why publiſh at all

all a work acknowledged ſo incomplete?" The author can only anſwer, that in the judgment of many reſpectable friends, the materials he had collected were too valuable to be thrown away; and that he could not ſuppoſe his work would be improved by *mere delay* of publication. And after all, he could not think his deficiencies extremely intereſting to the medical hiſtory of the period he has choſen. Of the more important printed works, ſeveral copies muſt be imagined to exiſt, all of which could ſcarcely eſcape a diligent ſearch continued for ſome years. He truſts it will appear that they have not; and that a tolerable idea may be formed of the ſtate of medicine and its practitioners, during a conſiderable portion of time, from the *memoirs* he has been able to compile.

SOME of the author's moſt eſteemed medical correſpondents have hinted a deſire

desire, that he would confine his researches to the progress of the *art*, without troubling himself with the *biography* of its *professors*. He is sensible that this is indeed the most useful and essential part of his undertaking; and he has, accordingly, by an account of every thing that seemed new and important in all the publications which came before him, attempted to fulfil this intention. But he could not persuade himself to forego the opportunities which offered of adding somewhat to the stock of *British Biography*; and of throwing due lustre on the characters of men, not less estimable for liberal manners and literary endowments, than for skill in their proper profession.

SHOULD this work be favoured with the public approbation and encouragement, the author may probably be induced to pursue the same plan

plan through ſucceeding periods, which preſent objects ſtill more intereſting, and leſs liable to deficiency in the execution. He has already made ſome advance in this deſign.

He concludes, with returning his grateful acknowledgments to thoſe Gentlemen who have forwarded his work, as well by their judicious advice, as by the books they have tranſmitted. If the performance he ventures to offer them, ſhall in any degree anſwer their expectations of information or amuſement, he doubts not but they will conſider themſelves as ſufficiently repaid.

CHRO-

CHRONOLOGICAL SERIES

OF

PERSONS OF WHOM MEMOIRS

ARE GIVEN IN THIS WORK.

	Born.	Flourished.	Died.
RICHARDUS ANGLICUS,	—	1230.	—
NICOLAS DE FERNEHAM,	—	—	1241.
JOHN GILES, or DE SANCTO ÆGIDIO,	—	13th. century.	—
HUGH OF EVESHAM,	—	—	1287.
GILBERTUS ANGLICUS,	—	end of 13th. cent.	—
JOHN OF GADDESDEN,	—	begin. of 14th. cent.	—
WILLIAM GRISAUNT,	—	an old man in 1350.	—
JOHN ARDERN,	—	1370.	—
JOHN MARFELDE,	—	begin. of 15th. cent.	—
NICHOLAS HOSTRESHAM,	—	1443.	—
JOHN PHREAS,	—	—	1465.
THOMAS LINACRE,	1460,	—	1524.
WILLIAM BUTTS,	—	—	1545.
JOHN CHAMBRE,	—	—	1549.
ANDREW BORDE,	—	—	1549.

	Born.	Flourished.	Died.
Edward Wotton,	1492.	—	1555.
Thomas Vicary,	—	1540.	—
George Owen,.	—	—	1558.
Robert Recorde,	—	—	1558.
Albayn Hyll,	—	—	1559.
Thomas Phayer,	—	—	1560.
Thomas Gibson,	—	—	1562.
William Turner,	—	—	1568.
John Clement,	—	—	1572.
Thomas Gale,	1507.	—	—
John Kaye, or Caius,	1510,	—	1573.
William Cuningham,	—	1559.	—
William Bulleyn,	—	—	1576.
Richard Caldwall,	—	—	1585.
John Securis,	—	1566.	—
George Etheridge,	1518.	—	—
John Jones,	—	1572.	—
George Baker,	—	1574.	—
John Banister,	—	1575.	—
Walter Baley,	1529,	—	1592.
Thomas Moufet,	—	—	about 1600.
John Halle,	1529.	—	—
John David Rhese,	1534,	—	1609.
William Butler,	1535,	—	1618.
William Gilbert,	1540,	—	1603.
William Clowes,	—	1573.	—
Peter Lowe,	—	—	1612.
Francis Anthony,	1550,	—	1623.
Richard Banister,	—	an old man in 1622.	
Matthew Gwinne,	—	—	1627.

Philemon

	Born.	Flourished.	Died.
Philemon Holland,	1551,	—	1636.
Theodore Goulston,	—	—	1632.
Edward Jorden,	1569,	—	1632.
John Woodall,	1569.	—	—
Theod. Turquet De Mayerne,	1573,	—	1655.
Robert Fludd,	1574,	—	1637.
Thomas Winston,	1575,	—	1655.
Tobias Venner,	1577,	—	1660.
William Harvey,	1578,	—	1658.
Francis Glisson,	1597,	—	1677.

E R R A T A.

Page 9, line ult. In following my authority too implicitly, I have not recollected that N. de Ferneham is said (p. 5.) to have been court physician to king Henry III.

P. 71, l. 7, *for* electoi *read* electio.

197, 5, *for* pharmacopea *read* pharmacopœia.

222, 18 and 21, *for* pharmacopœa *read* pharmacopœia.

INTRODUCTION.

THE Hiſtory of Medicine and of Medical Practitioners in this iſland during thoſe dark ages which ſo long overſhadowed the countries of Europe, affords very little to intereſt the curioſity of thoſe who have not already acquired the habit of valuing antiquity for its own ſake. At a period when all merit, even in the moſt celebrated ſchools of phyſic, conſiſted in underſtanding and commenting upon the fanciful reveries of Arabian writers, who debaſed all the knowledge they had received from purer ſources, what improvements could be expected among the ignorant and illiterate profeſſors of a country, remote from the centre of ſcience, and ſunk in barbariſm beyond its neighbours? Or what biographical memoirs, either inſtructive or amuſing, can be collected from the obſcure accounts of perſons void of all ſpirit of rational enquiry, and untinctured with the elegancies of polite literature?

THE learned and ingenious Dr. Freind has, indeed, thought it worth while in his *Hiſtory of Phyſick* to give a view of ſome of the writings ſtill extant of our earlieſt medical anceſtors, by way of ſpecimens of the doctrines and practice of the times. This he has done in ſo judicious and agreeable a manner, that it would be equally preſumptuous and unneceſſary to attempt executing it after him. To his well-known work, therefore, I refer for information as far as his plan leads him; contenting myſelf with mentioning as the general reſult, that the greateſt part of their writings, particularly all the *rationale* of diſeaſes, was a compilation from the Arabians and their copyiſts; and that the reſt conſiſted of a heterogeneous collection of receipts and directions

directions, drawn from the copious stores of empiricism and superstition.

SOME accounts of the lives of several other early practitioners and writers, whose works are not come down to us, are extant in the memoirs of our literary biographers, Leland, Pits, and Bale. These, though very jejune and dry, are yet worthy of a perusal, as serving to give the best insight into the education, character and course of studies of physicians in those ages. I shall therefore select from the above writers such of these articles as may sufficiently answer the purpose of the present *Introduction*; which is, to give a general idea of the state of physic in these countries, till the dawning of a more enlightened period, which will offer more valuable and interesting objects to our enquiries.

THE first English medical writer recorded by these authors is named

RICHARDUS ANGLICUS. He flourished about the year 1230. He is said to have studied first at Oxford, and then at

 Paris.

Paris. As a proof of his general reputation we find him mentioned by Simphorianus Champerius in his treatise on medical writers, as one of the most eminent of his profession. The following ample list of his works is given.

De Crisi.
Summa de criticis diebus.
De Pulsibus.
De Modo conficiendi & medendi.
Tractatus de urinis.
De Regulis urinarum.
De Signis morborum.
De Signis prognosticis.
De Phlebotomia.
Anatomia, Galeni more.
Correctorium Alchimiæ.
De Febribus.
Speculum Alchimiæ.
De Re medica.
Repressiva.
De Signis febrium.

LELAND says he wrote other works, which were not preserved.

NICOLAS DE FERNEHAM was educated at Oxford, where, we are told, he exhibited early proofs of uncommon genius, and attained to great proficiency in the learning of the age. Having a particular inclination to botany and physic, he pursued these studies, first at Paris, and then at Bologna, under the best masters; and applied diligently to the works

works of Hippocrates, Galen, and Dioſcorides. After a long abſence, he returned to England, and was held in high eſtimation both as a phyſician and a ſcholar. He was called to court by King Henry III. and entertained as his domeſtic phyſician at a large ſalary. At length, when (as Pits obſerves) the good old man was entirely attached to reading the ſcriptures, and meditating on ſpiritual things, after having refuſed the ſee of Cheſter, he was made biſhop of Durham, by the intereſt of Otho, the pope's legate. In this city he died in the year 1241. Matthew Paris mentions him with particular applauſe. His medical works were, *Practicæ Medicinæ*, lib. I. *De viribus herbarum*, lib. I. and ſeveral others of which the titles are not recorded.

JOHN GILES, in Latin JOANNES ÆGIDIUS, or *de* SANCTO ÆGIDIO, was born at St. Alban's, and flouriſhed in the thirteenth century. He was educated at Paris, and became phyſician in ordinary to Philip king of France, and a profeſſor of medicine in the univerſities of Paris and Montpellier. He was afterwards created a doctor of divinity, and was the first Englishman who entered among the Dominicans, with whom he became a celebrated preacher. In his old age he was famous for his divinity lectures at Oxford. Matthew Paris relates, that Robert Grosthead, the famous bishop of Lincoln, lying on his death-bed, sent for Master John Giles, learned in physic and divinity, that he might receive comfort from him both for body and soul. This prelate died in 1253; and it is probable Giles was of an advanced age at that time.

He left behind him two medical pieces, entitled *Practicæ Medicinales* and *Futurorum Prognostica*; some commentaries on Aristotle; and a number of theological treatises.

HUGH of EVESHAM, or HUGO ATRATUS, was born at Evesham in Worcestershire. After perfecting himself in philosophy, mathematics, and the other liberal arts in both our English universities, he travelled through all the celebrated seminaries of learning in France and Italy in pursuit of medical knowledge, In this he made so great a proficiency,

ficiency, as to become, we are told, the firſt of his profeſſion, not only in his own country, but of the age he lived in, which was the thirteenth century. He was alſo very eminent for mathematical and aſtronomical knowledge; and according to the cuſtom of the age, united the clerical character with the medical, being a prebendary in the cathedral of York, procurator for the archbiſhop of York at the court of Rome, an archdeacon of Worceſter, and rector of Spofford in the dioceſe of York. In conſequence of his high reputation, he was ſent for to Rome in the year 1280, by pope Martin IV. to aſſiſt in the deciſion of certain newly promulgated and difficult queſtions in phyſic. What theſe were, we are not informed; however, our countryman acquitted himſelf ſo much to the ſatisfaction of the court of Rome, and excited ſo great an admiration of his learning, that the pope, in the year 1281, created him a cardinal prieſt, by the ſtyle of Cardinal of St. Laurence in Lucina. From that time he applied himſelf ſolely to theological ſtudies; and at length, in the year 1287, he died of the plague with ſeveral other cardinals in the conclave held after the death of pope Honorius IV. Bale, who ſeldom allows a pope or cardinal to die a natural death, ſays he was poiſoned; and this report is alſo adopted in in the *Annal. Vigorn.* Pits relates that many important remains of this perſon were extant in his time at Rome, eſpecially in the church of St. Laurence, or Lorenzo, in Lucina, where he was buried, and a ſplendid monument erected for him. He was a benefactor to this church, as appears from the following paſſage in the *Roma antica e moderna, tom. I. p.* 434, under the deſcription of this edifice. "Ugo Cardinal Ingleſe, e Innico Avalos, Spagnuolo, ſuoi titolari, gli fecero in diverſi tempi vari riſtori ed abbellimenti."

He is ſaid to have publiſhed the following works.

Super opere febrium Iſaac. Problemata quædam. Medicinales canones. De Genealogiis humanis.

GILBERTUS ANGLICUS is placed by Bale (who calls him *Gilbertus Legleus,* and ſays he was phyſician to Hubert, archbiſhop of of Canterbury) in the reign of king John, about the year 1210. But Leland makes him more modern; and from ſome paſſages in his writings it appears that he muſt have flouriſhed towards the end of the thirteenth century. The memoirs of his life are very ſcanty; and he is chiefly known as the author of a *Compendium of phyſic*, ſtill extant, and which is the earlieſt remaining writing on the practice of medicine among our countrymen. This is one of the books commented on by Dr. Freind; who, with great impartiality, while he is obliged to take off ſomewhat from the high character given of the author by Leland, yet allows him a ſhare of merit which may place him on a level with the medical writers of that age. To Dr. Freind's Hiſtory I refer for the particulars worthy of notice in Gilbert's works; as likewiſe for the very entertaining and well-written account of

JOHN OF GADDESDEN, author of the famous *Roſa Anglica*. He flouriſhed towards the beginning of the fourteenth century, and ſeems to have had very extenſive and lucrative practice; and was the firſt Engliſhman who was employed as a phyſician at court. The ignorance, ſuperſtition and low quackery which appear throughout his practice, and which are painted with much life and humour by Freind, do no great honour to the character of the profeſſion in that age, and ſhew with how much abatement we are to take the high-flown panegyricks contained in the accounts of our biographers. On peruſing the *Roſa Anglica*, I found one paſſage not noticed by Freind, which may be worth attention. My readers will probably be ſurpriſed to find that the method of producing freſh from ſalt water by ſimple diſtillation ſhould be familiarly mentioned by an author of this remote period. In a chapter of John of Gaddeſden's on ſweetning ſalt water, he gives the four following methods of performing it. 1ſt. Repeated percolation through ſand. 2dly. Boiling ſalt water in an open veſſel, and receiving the ſteam on a cloth, which, when ſufficiently impregnated, is to be wrung out. (This, in fact, is a kind of diſtillation.) 3dly. *Diſtillation in an alembic with a gentle heat.* 4thly. Setting a thin cup of wax to ſwim in a veſſel of ſalt water, when the ſweet water

water will drain through the pores of the wax, and be received in the cup.*

I SHALL only further obſerve concerning this perſon, that though he undoubtedly devoted himſelf to the practice of his profeſſion, he poſſeſſed the prebend of St. Paul's in the ſtall of Ealdland. It ſeems probable from this and other inſtances, that the procurement of a ſinecure place in the church was a method in which the great ſometimes paid the ſervices of their phyſicians.

WILLIAM GRISAUNT purſued his philoſophical ſtudies in Merton college, Oxford; where by plunging into the depths of mathematics and aſtronomy, he excited a violent ſuſpicion, as fryar Bacon had done before him, of being engaged in magical practices. It was probably on this account that, when arrived at years of maturity, he went into France, where he devoted himſelf entirely to the ſtudy of medicine, firſt at Montpellier, and then at Marſeilles. In this latter city

* *Roſa Anglic.* fol. 135.

he

he fixed his refidence, and lived by the practice of his profeffion, in which he acquired great fkill and eminence. He is faid affiduoufly to have purfued the method inftituted by the Greek phyficians, of inveftigating the nature and caufe of the difeafe, and the conftitution of the patient; from which, and from the fufpicions he laboured under in the earlier part of life, we may conclude him to have been of a genius fuperior to his time. We are told that he was an old man in 1350; and that he had a fon who was firft an abbot of canons regular at Marfeilles, and at length arrived at the pontificate under the name of Urban V.

THE following lift is given of Grifaunt's works.

Speculum Aftrologiæ.	*De Motu capitis.*
De Qualitatibus aftrorum.	*De Caufa ignorantiæ.*
De Magnitudine folis.	*De Urina non vifa.*
De Quadratura circuli.	*De Judicio patientis.*
De Significationibus eorundem.	

JOHN ARDERN is another of our early writers whofe works come within the notice of of Dr. Freind. I ſhall therefore only mention that he was a Surgeon of great experience, and the firſt who is recorded as having become eminent in that branch among our countrymen—that his reſidence was in the town of Newark, from the year 1348 to 1370, when he removed to London, whither his reputation had long before reached—and that although a great mixture of empiriciſm and ſuperſtition appears in his practice, yet ſeveral uſeful obſervations are to be found in his writings, and he may be reckoned among thoſe who have really improved their profeſſion. A treatiſe of his on the *Fiſtula in Ano* was thought worthy of being tranſlated and publiſhed by John Read in 1588.

Dr. Freind remarks, that it appears from Ardern to have been the cuſtom of the times for ſecurity to be required by ſurgeons from their patients for payment when the cure was effected. I ſhall obſerve on this head that the ſame thing was practiſed in France at the beginning of the preſent century; for we are told, in the *eloge* of Monſieur Mareſchal, in the *Memoirs of the Royal Academy of Surgery*

at

at Paris, that when he was appointed first surgeon to Louis XIV. in 1703, he generously threw into the fire obligatory bonds from his patients to the value of 20,000 livres.

JOHN MARFELDE was educated at Oxford, and settled in the practice of his profession in London, of which city he was a native. He is said to have flourished in the reign of Henry VI. He was in great fame both for learning and medical skill; and wrote several treatises in physic, one of which only was extant in the time of Bale and Pits, entitled *Praxis Medicinæ*. This was composed in imitation of the work of Gilbertus Anglicus; and the character given of it is, that though inferior to Gilbert's in the speculative, it was greatly superior in the practical part.

NICHOLAS HOSTRESHAM flourished about the year 1443, and is, from his name, supposed by Fuller to have been a native of Horsham in Sussex. He is said to have been a very eminent physician, and in high esteem among

among the nobility as well for his conversation as his medical skill. He wrote several books, of which the following list is given.

Viaticorum necessariorum, lib. VII.
Antidotarium, lib. I.
Contra dolorem renum, lib. I.
De Febribus, lib. I.
Practicæ medicinæ, lib. I.
De Modo conficiendi & dispensandi, lib. I.
Besides others, the titles of which are lost.

I CANNOT better conclude this short view of the state of physic and its practitioners among us at what may be called its barbarous period, than by presenting to the reader the character of a *doctor of physic* as drawn by a cotemporary poet, remarkable for his natural and lively descriptions. Chaucer, in the *Prologue* to his *Canterbury Tales*, among the various personages who compose the respectable company of pilgrims at the sign of the Taberde, introduces a physician, whom he thus characterizes. (It is to be observed that this pilgrimage is supposed to have happened in the year 1364.)

THE

THE DOCTOR OF PHYSIK.

With us there was a Doctor of Physik,
In al the worldé was ther non hym lyk,
To speke of Physik and of Surgerye;
For he was groundit in Astronomy.
He kept his pacient a ful gret del
In hourys by his Magyk Naturel;
Wel couth he fortunen the ascendent
Of his ymagys for his pacient.
He knew the cause of every maladye,
Were it or hot or cold, or moist or drye,
Where they engendere, and of what humour.
He was a veray parfyt practysour.
The cause yknowe, and of his harm the rote,
Anon he yaf (1) to the syk man his bote. (2)

Full redy had he his Apothecaryes,
To sendyn him his droggis, and letewaryes, (3)
For eche of hem made other for to wynne,
Her (4) frenschepe was not nowé to begynne.

Wel knew he the old *Esculapius*,
And *Dioscordes*, and eke *Rufus*,

1. Gave. 2. Remedy. 3. Electuaries. 4. Their.

Old

Old *Hyppocras*, *Lylye*, and *Galien*,
Serapion, *Razis*, and *Avycen*,
Averois, *Damaſcyen*, and *Conſtantyn*,
Bernard, and *Gadeſleun*, and *Gilbertyn*.

Of his diete meſurable was he,
For it was non of ſuperfluite,
But of gret nuryſchynge, and digeſtible:
His ſtudy was but lytyl in the bible.
In ſanguyn(5) and in perſe(6) he clad was al
Lined with taffata and with ſendal;(7)
And yit he was but eſy of diſpence,
He kepté that he won in peſtelence;
For gold in phyſik is a cordial;
Therefore he lovede gold in ſpecial.

A FEW remarks on this curious portrait may not be unintereſting.

THIS Doctor is repreſented as qualified to ſpeak of ſurgery as well as phyſic; though the practice of it was a ſeparate branch then as

5. Blood-colour. 6. A bluiſh-grey, or ſky-colour. 7. A fine ſilken ſtuff.

well as now, as we know by the example of the celebrated ſurgeon Ardern, who flouriſhed at this very time.

The fundamental ſcience on which his knowledge was built is ſaid to be *Aſtronomy*; by which is underſtood that fanciful part of it, chiefly, which we now term Aſtrology. By the aſſiſtance of this, he was enabled to make election of fortunate hours for the adminiſtration of his remedies, and to calculate the nativities of his patients, in order to diſcover which of the heavenly bodies was lord of the aſcendant at their birth; and likewiſe, by *magic natural*, to make ſigils or characters ſtamped in metal, with the ſignature of that conſtellation which governed the part of the body where the diſeaſe was ſeated.

His reaſonings concerning the cauſes of diſtempers were founded on the Galenical doctrines of the four different qualities of heat, cold, dryneſs, and moiſture, operáting on the different humours of the body.

As

As well as his modern brethren he had his apothecaries under him, who furnifhed him with his *drugs* and *electuaries*; that is, his fimples and compounds, the moft noted of which laft clafs were in the form of electuaries.

Among the mafters from whom he derived the principles of his art, we find the venerable father of phyfic; fome of the elder Greeks; feveral of the Arabian fchool; the modern Greeks, Damafcenus Prefbyter, and Conftantine the Monk; Raymond Lully (called here Lylye;) Bernard de Gordonio, author of the celebrated *Lilium Medicinæ*; and his own countrymen, Gilbert and Gaddefden.

From the farcafm thrown out concerning his unacquaintance with the fcriptures, we may judge that he did not, like many of that and an earlier age, unite the clerical with the medical character; and from the defcription of his drefs and equipment, we may conclude him to have been a perfon of fome figure and dignity. Upon the whole, with respect to the manner of conducting the business of his profession, and the rank he occupied in society, he appears to have approached nearer to the same character in modern times than might have been imagined.

BIOGRA-

BIOGRAPHICAL

MEMOIRS OF MEDICINE

IN GREAT BRITAIN

FROM THE REVIVAL OF LITERATURE.

IT is impoffible exactly to mark out the commencement of fuch a period as that of the revival of literature. Several gradual fteps led in fucceffion to this defirable event; and the proportional advance towards it was much greater in fome countries than in others. In Italy there exifted elegant writers formed on the beft models of the antients, at a time when all the reft of Europe was funk in barbarifm. If any one circumftance, however, may be pointed out as peculiarly inftrumental in propagating liberal and uſeful learning throughout the weſtern world, it is perhaps that of the taking of Conſtantinople by the Turks in the year 1453, which occaſioned the diſperſion of ſeveral learned men ſkilled in the Greek language, who carried their knowledge and their books to their places of refuge. Accordingly, we find ſoon after this period a number of tranſlations of the Greek authors, as well medical as others, undertaken by the literati of various countries. Medicine gained by this very eſſentially, as it was freed from the mixture of Arabian folly and extravagance by a direct application to the purer ſources of the Greeks. And its profeſſors were not leſs benefited by the acquiſition of thoſe ornamental parts of literature, which diſpelled the barbariſm of their language, and formed that union of the character of the polite ſcholar with that of the phyſician, which they have ever ſince, ſo much to their credit, maintained.

IT is generally imagined that the celebrated *Linacre* was the firſt of our countrymen in whom this combination ſubſiſted; but great as his merit was in this reſpect, we cannot without injuſtice overlook the claims of an earlier ornament of the profeſſion, concerning whom, indeed, our memoirs are leſs copious than might be wiſhed. This was

JOHN PHREAS

TO whom Leland gives his teſtimony in the following words. "Is ex numero Anglo-"rum primus mihi quidem eſſe videatur, qui "barbarie patriam fæde gravatam labore "honeſto, atque adeo utili, plane valetudini "priſtinæ, qua imperantibus Romanis ſupra "hominum opinionem omnem floruit, inte-"gre reſtituit." From this author's account of his life the enſuing memoirs are collected,

JOHN PHREAS was born in London at the end of the 14th, or beginning of the 15th century. He was educated at Oxford, and became fellow of Balliol college. Having taken holy orders, he was ſettled at Briſtol by means of a friend, as miniſter of St. Mary's church on the mount in that city. In this ſituation he continued to purſue with the greateſt ardour the literary ſtudies for which he had made himſelf famous at the univerſity. At length, being informed by ſome merchants trading from Briſtol to Italy, of the number of ingenious men then flouriſhing in that ſeat of the Muſes, he determined to viſit it; and as ſoon as he had collected a ſum of money for his ſupport, he ſet ſail for that country. Guarini was then a famous teacher of philoſophy at Ferrara. Phreas attended his lectures, and at the ſame time attached himſelf to the ſtudies of civil law and medicine. In the latter ſcience he proceeded ſo far as himſelf to lecture publickly at Ferrara, with a great reſort of learned men. He afterwards did the ſame at Florence and Padua, in which laſt univerſity he was preſented with the degree of Doctor of Phyſic in a very reſpectful manner. From thence he went to Rome; and in that city diſplayed his medical and literary abilities with great reputation. John Tiptoft, Earl of Worceſter, was then at Rome, having taken refuge there from the civil commotions which were at that time raging in England between the houſes of York and Lancaſter. This nobleman was educated

educated at Balliol college together with Phreas; and was the only English person of quality who patronized learning in that period. He honoured Phreas with very particular marks of favour at Rome, who in return dedicated several of his works to him.

THE extraordinary merit of Phreas attracted the notice of pope Paul II; and in return for his dedicating to him a translation of Diodorus Siculus, that pontiff created him bishop of Bath and Wells. This advancement, however, he did not live to enjoy; dying at Rome before consecration, in 1465, not without suspicion of being poisoned by a competitor. He is said to have left behind him a large fortune, acquired in Italy by the practice of physic.

PHREAS appears to have been a master of both the learned languages. His works are chiefly of the light and elegant kind. Leland mentions having read a copy of very harmonious verses, in which he makes Bacchus expostulate with a goat for browzing the tender vines. They were dedicated to the Earl of Worcefter. The fubject of another little piece is *De coma parvi facienda.* A circumftance perhaps more to his credit than any other, is that he was requefted by a noble Italian to write an epitaph for the tomb of Petrarch, to fupply the place of a barbarous one before infcribed upon it. When the partiality of that nation for their favourite, and one whofe extraordinary reputation had done them fo much honour, is confidered, it muft feem a high compliment to a foreigner to be entrufted with the charge of tranfmitting his memory to pofterity in the infcription on his monument. Leland mentions this piece as in his poffeffion. He wrote, befides, feveral poems on various occafions, epiftles, and epigrams. Alfo, a treatife on *Geography*; another on *Cofmography* (collected from Pliny;) and one entitled *Contra Diodorum Siculum poeticé fabulantem.* He tranflated from the Greek into Latin

Xenophontis quædam, lib. fex.
Diodori Siculi bibliotheca, lib. fex.
Sinefius de calvitio, lib. unus.

THIS

THIS laſt was printed at Baſil in 1521. Part of the dedication to the Earl of Worceſter, is quoted by Leland in his account of that nobleman: it is the only ſpecimen of his writings I have met with; and gives a very favourable idea of his Latin ſtyle. I find from a note of the ingenious and learned Mr. Warton, in his *Hiſtory of Engliſh Poetry*, vol. II. p. 423, that ſome Epiſtles of Phreas are ſtill extant in M. S. in the library of Baliol College and the Bodleian. Among theſe is one to his preceptor Guarini; whoſe epiſtles are full of encomiums on Phreas. Five are written from Italy to his fellow-ſtudent and patron Gray, biſhop of Ely. In one he complains that the biſhop's remittances of money had failed, and that he was obliged to pawn his books and cloaths to Jews at Ferrara. Theſe letters, Mr. Warton ſays, "diſcover an uncommon terſeneſs and facility of expreſſion."

PHREAS muſt be regarded as a premature production of Engliſh literature, foſtered by the kindly influence of a more favourable climate; in which, indeed, he paſſed the greater

greater part of his life. It is not ſurpriſing, therefore, that he had no immediate ſucceſſors in his native country; and that the buſineſs of introducing a laſting reformation into the character of the Engliſh phyſician was reſerved for the ſubject of our next article, after the intervention of a conſiderable number of years.

THOMAS LINACRE.

WAS born at the city of Canterbury in or about the year 1460. He was deſcended from the family of Linacres of Linacre-hall near Cheſterfield in Derbyſhire; whence Fuller and others have been led into the miſtake of ſuppoſing Derby the place of his birth. He was educated at Canterbury under an eminent ſchoolmaſter named William Tilly, or De Selling; and from thence removed to Oxford, where he was choſen fellow of All-Soul's college in 1484. His deſire of further advancement in learning incited him to travel into Italy; aud he accordingly accompanied his former

former maſter De Selling, who was appointed ambaſſador from Henry VII. to the court of Rome. De Selling left Linacre at Bologna under the care of his old friend Angelo Politian, with the moſt particular recommendations. This perſon was at that time accounted one of the moſt polite ſcholars and elegant Latiniſts in Europe; yet our young ſtudent by his aſſiduous application attained a greater purity of ſtyle in that language than Politian himſelf. At Florence, Linacre was ſo fortunate as to acquire the favour of the Duke Lorenzo de Medicis, a prince of great affability, and a munificent patron of literature; who granted him permiſſion to attend the ſame preceptors with his own ſons. Here he had the opportunity of perfecting himſelf in Greek under Demetrius Chalcondylas, a refugee from Conſtantinople at the time of its being taken by the Turks.

THUS accompliſhed in claſſical learning, he went to Rome, and applied himſelf to the ſtudy of medicine and natural philoſophy under Hermolaus Barbarus; and is ſaid to have been the firſt Engliſhman who underſtood

ſtood Ariſtotle and Galen in the original Greek. He tranſlated many pieces of the latter author with great elegance, as we ſhall mention more at large hereafter; and in conjunction with Grocyn and Latimer, his illuſtrious collegues in the advancement of ancient learning, undertook a tranſlation of the former, which, however, was left imperfect. On his return, he took the degree of doctor of phyſic at Oxford, and was made public profeſſor of medicine; or, rather, read lectures *gratis* in that faculty. He likewiſe taught the Greek language in the univerſity. His reputation was, however, too great to ſuffer him long to continue in this ſituation; and he was called to court by king Henry VII, who entruſted him with the care both of the health and education of his ſon prince Arthur. We are likewiſe told that he was teacher of the Italian language to this prince and the princeſs Catharine. He was made ſucceſſively phyſician to the kings Henry VII. Henry VIII. and Edward VI. and the princeſs Mary.

In this exalted ſtation he was not forgetful of the intereſts of his profeſſion, and of mankind

kind in general. Befides founding two lectureſhips of phyſic at Oxford, and one at Cambridge, he projected and accompliſhed a moſt important ſervice to medicine by the inſtitution of the *Royal College of Phyſicians in London.* He had beheld with concern the practice of this moſt uſeful art chiefly engroſſed by illiterate monks, and empirics; a natural conſequence of committing the power of approving and licenſing practitioners to the biſhops in their ſeveral dioceſes, who certainly muſt, in general, have been very incompetent judges of medical ability. To ſtrike at the root of this evil, he therefore obtained, by his intereſt with cardinal Wolſey, letters patent from Henry VIII, dated in the year 1518, conſtituting a corporate body of regular bred phyſicians in London, in whom ſhould reſide the ſole privilege of admitting perſons to practice within that city, and a circuit of ſeven miles round it; and alſo of licenſing practitioners throughout the whole kingdom, except ſuch as were graduates of Oxford or Cambridge, who by virtue of their degrees were independent of the college except within London and its precincts. The

college

college had likewiſe authority to examine preſcriptions and the drugs in apothecaries ſhops; and their cenſures were enforced with the power of inflicting fines and impriſonment. The letters patent are ſaid to be granted at the requeſt of the following perſons; John Chambre, Thomas Linacre, and Fernandus de Victoria, phyſicians to the king; Nicholas Halſwell, John Fraunces, and Robert Yaxley, phyſicians; and cardinal Wolſey. Linacre was the firſt preſident of the new college, and continued in that office during the remainder of his life. Its aſſemblies were held at his houſe in Knight-Rider's ſtreet, which he bequeathed to the college at his death.

Towards the latter part of his life, in the year 1519, Linacre entered into holy orders; the motives to which ſtep are not a little dubious. If, as ſome aſſert, the only benefice conferred upon him was a chantorſhip in the cathedral of York, it would be moſt obvious to ſuppoſe that a ſuperſtitious regard to the clerical character was his chief inducement. But others mention his appointment to ſeveral other

other church preferments ; none of them, however, very profitable; and moſt of them reſigned ſoon after his induction to them. From a paſſage in an epiſtle of his to Warham, archbiſhop of Canterbury, it would ſeem that the acquiſition of an eaſy and honourable retreat had been his principal object. "Statu-"eram, ampliſſime Præſul, pro ocio, in quod "me honorifico collato ſacerdotio ex negocio "primus vindicaſti, merito primos ejus fructus "tibi dedicare." It appears that about this time he was exceedingly afflicted with that painful diſeaſe which at length put an end to his life, and muſt now have greatly incapacitated him from buſineſs. Whatever his motives were, it is ſaid, however, that on the aſſumption of this new character he applied himſelf to thoſe ſtudies which are more peculiarly connected with it; and to this purpoſe a remarkable anecdote is told by Sir John Cheke. He relates, that Linacre, a little before his death, when worn out with ſickneſs and fatigues, firſt began to read the New Teſtament; and that when he had peruſed the fifth, ſixth, and ſeventh chapters of St. Matthew, he threw the book from him with great violence, paſſionately exclaiming, "either this is not the goſpel, or we are not chriſtians!"—a declaration, if rightly underſtood, equally honourable to the morals he found there inculcated, and ſatirical to thoſe of the age. It is, nevertheleſs, agreed on all hands that the character of this eminent perſon, whether as an upright and humane phyſician, a ſteady and affectionate friend, or a munificent patron of letters, was deſerving of the higheſt applauſe. Were other teſtimonies wanting, it were ſufficient in juſtification of this eulogium to mention that he was the intimate friend of Eraſmus. That great and worthy man frequently takes occaſion to expreſs his affection and eſteem for his character and abilities; and writing to an acquaintance, when taken ill at Paris, he pathetically laments his abſence from Linacre, from whoſe ſkill and kindneſs he might receive equal relief. We find from another letter of Eraſmus that he afterwards imagined himſelf injured by Linacre; but, with much generoſity, he declares he ſhall oppoſe to this one injury the many benefits he had received from him.

Linacre died, in great agonies from the ſtone, October 20, 1524, aged 64; and was buried in St. Paul's Cathedral, where a monument was afterwards erected to his memory by his admirer and ſucceſſor in fame, Dr. Caius.

Having thus gone through all the important occurrences of the life of this eminent phyſician, which have been tranſmitted to poſterity, I ſhall beſtow a particular conſideration on his literary character, as ſo intimately connected with the annals of learning, in an age memorable for the revival of it. And this method of ſeparating the biographical from the critical part of theſe memoirs I ſhall generally follow, for the ſake of a more diſtinct view of each of theſe objects.

The advantages this perſon received in his education ſeem to have been not a little uncommon in that age; for Eraſmus, reciting the names of many of the moſt eminent phyſicians in Europe who ſtudied the Greek language in their declining years, mentions Linacre and Ruellius as the only perſons of their profeſſion who had had the good fortune to ſtudy it when young. Tranſlations from the Greek authors into Latin were indeed the chief occupations of the literati of thoſe times, and ſeveral of the Italian ſcholars had employed their pens in theſe uſeful works; but no Engliſhman except Phreas ſeems to have undertaken this difficult taſk, at leaſt with ſucceſs, before Linacre. His firſt eſſay was a tranſlation of *Proclus on the Sphere*, concerning which, Eraſmus gives the following relation: that it was dedicated to king Henry VII.; but that Bernard Andreas, tutor to prince Arthur, maliciouſly inſinuated to the king that the book had been tranſlated before (as indeed it had, but in a wretched manner); whence his majeſty was ſo highly diſguſted, as to contemn the offering, and ever after to entertain an extreme averſion for Linacre. In this account, however, there is a miſtake, as the book was dedicated to his pupil prince Arthur. It was printed in 1499 by Aldus Manutius, with a recommendatory preface by that learned man.

But our author's literary reputation was principally raiſed by his tranſlations from Galen;

Galen; in which he not only ſhewed a laudable attachment to the improvement of his profeſſion, but exhibited a Latin ſtyle ſo pure and elegant, as ranked him among the fineſt writers of his age. The talent of compoſing in correct and claſſical Latin was at that time an object of more peculiar emulation than perhaps it has ever been ſince; and our phyſician ſeems to have been ſcrupulouſly attentive, even beyond moſt of his cotemporaries, to arrive at perfection in this point. Eraſmus ſummarily deſcribes him "Vir non exacti tantum, ſed ſeveri judicii;" and in one of his epiſtles thus gently reprehends his exceſſive delicacy. "At tu, ſi mihi "permittis ut liberé tecum agam, ſine fine "premis tuas omnium eruditiſſimas lucubra-"tiones, ut periculum ſit ne pro cauto mo-"deſtoque crudelis habearis, qui ſtudia hujus "ſeculi tam lenta torqueas expectatione tuo-"rum laborum." The learned Huet in his treatiſe *De claris Interpretatoribus* gives a ſimilar judgment. "Adeamus Thomam Lina-"crum, quo nemo majorem orationis nito-"rem, caſtitatem, & condecentiam ad inter-"pretationem contulit: quarum virtutum in-"tegritatem dum diligentius tueri ſtudet,

 fidelem

" fidelem verborum affectationem, raro qui-" dem, at aliquando tamen, omisit." In the famous controversy concerning Ciceronianism, so warmly agitated among the scholars of that age, Erasmus characterized many eminent authors, both antient and modern, in his celebrated dialogue entitled *Ciceronianus*. Speaking of Linacre, he thus describes his manner of writing, with a particular reference to the author in question. " Novi (Linacrum) vi-" rum undequaque doctissimum, sed sic affec-" tum erga Ciceronem, ut etiamsi potuisset " utrumlibet, prius habuisset esse Quintiliano " similis quam Ciceroni, non ita multo in " hunc æquior quam est Græcorum vulgus. " Urbanitatem nusquam affectat, ab affectibus " abstinet religiosius quam ullus Atticus, bre-" viloquentiam et elegantiam amat, ad do-" cendum intentus. Aristotelem & Quintili-" anum studuit exprimere. Huic igitur viro " per me quantum voles laudum tribuas li-" cebit; Tullianus dici non potest, qui stu-" duerit Tullio esse dissimilis." Sir John Cheke, who in other instances has shewn somewhat of an unfriendly spirit towards Linacre, may be thought not uninfluenced by it

in

in the following account of his literary character, though interſperſed with due commendations. " Fecit in Medicina tantum, " quantum alius Latinus illius ætatis quiſ" quam. Et quamdiu in Medicina ſe conti" net, tamdiu laudem ſingularem habet: ſin " foras ſerpat, & Oratores carpat, videat ne " ultra crepidam progrediatur. Nam quan" quam in transferendis Galeni libris, laus " ejus eſt prope ſingularis: tamen ſi de acu" mine & celeritate ingenii diſputatur, aut de " rebus popularibus graviter & diſerte trac" tandis, in eo, ſi nunc viveret, aliis laudem " concederet, Medicinam ipſe aſſumeret. Et " tamen cur tam faſtidioſus eſſet in audiendo " Cicerone, neſcio. Illud videmus, omnes " quos ille libros *De Latini ſermonis ſtructura* " compoſuit, exemplis Ciceronis abundare: " ut non tam fortaſſe neglexerit, quam animi " quadam moroſitate videri voluit neglexiſſe."

De pronunc. Græc.

The firſt piece of Galen of which Linacre publiſhed a tranſlation, was his treatiſe *De tuenda ſanitate*, in ſix books. He ſays he was encouraged to offer this to the public by the persuasions of several of the most learned men in Italy, Germany and France, and particularly Erasmus and Budæus. It was printed at Cambridge in 1517, and dedicated to king Henry VIII. as was likewise his translation of the fourteen books *De morbis curandis*, printed at Paris in 1526. The three books *De temperamentis*, and one *De inæquali temperie* appeared first at Cambridge in 1521; they were inscribed to Pope Leo X. The three books *De naturalibus facultatibus* which he mentions in an epistle to archbishop Warham, as designed to be dedicated to him, were, according to Mattaire, reprinted by Colinæus in 1528, together with one book *De pulsuum usu* from Galen, and some remarks of Paulus Ægineta *De diebus criticis*. I cannot find when or where these were first printed. In the same year our author's posthumous translation of Galen's four books *De symptomatibus* was printed by Colinæus, who also reprinted all his other translations.

Our learned physician was no less distinguished as a most accurate grammarian. Besides a small book of the rudiments of the Latin

Latin grammar, written in Englifh for the ufe of the princefs Mary, and afterwards tranflated into Latin by the celebrated Buchanan, he publifhed a larger work entitled *De emendata ftructura Latini fermonis, libri fex.** This

* I HAVE been favoured by a gentleman of great learning and judgment with the following character of this piece: which I infert, not only as an honourable teftimony in favour of our author, but as a means to recall in fome meafure the attention of fcholars to a work which has fallen into an unmerited neglect.

"THIS treatife is introduced by a recommendatory letter of Melanchton, a man not only eminent as a polemic divine, but likewife juftly celebrated for his elegant and claffic tafte. He fpeaks of the work before us as inferior to none of it's kind then extant; and (notwithftanding the multitude of Latin grammars that have been fince written) were he living at this time he would not perhaps think it neceffary to make many exceptions. Linacre appears by this work to have been well acquainted with the ancient grammarians, Greek and Latin; writers who appear, from the ufe made of them by the elegant and learned author of Hermes, not to have deferved that neglect they have long lain under. This treatife muft not however be confidered as a mere compilation from former grammars; for the author appears to have thought much and deeply on the fubject himfelf. There

This was universally acknowledged to be a work of the most profound erudition; and indeed it appears to have engaged a portion of his time and attention, almost too great, with regard to the other more important occupations of his profession and station. This at

There are many just remarks applicable to language in general; but the substance of the book relates, as its title denotes, to the Latin tongue in particular, of which he seems to have had the most accurate knowledge. His work is divided into six books: the two first treat of *Analogy*, the remaining four of *Syntax*. His observations and rules are expressed with brevity and plainness, in the purest Latin, and illustrated by well chosen examples from the most approved writers. As he has treated his subject in its full extension, he will be thought by some to have used too many divisions and subdivisions, and to have overburthened the art of grammar with a multitude of unnecessary mechanical terms. This is indeed contrary to the present mode of teaching, which is calculated to make literature as easy and common as possible, that all persons may be, or at least appear to be, skilled in any part of learning, without the loss of much time, or the exertion of much labour. A more superficial way of writing, and such as requires few terms of art, is no doubt best adapted to this purpose; but let it be remembered, that it is impossible to go deep in any art or science without a great number of such. Nor let it be thought that at leaſt was the opinion of Eraſmus, who in his *Moriæ encomium* expoſes his friend, not indeed by name, but by ſufficiently obvious marks, in the following good-natured banter. "Novi quendam πολυτεχνοτατον, Græcum, La-"tinum, Mathematicum, Philoſophum, Me-"dicum, και ταυτα βαςιλικον, jam ſexagenarium, "qui cæteris rebus omiſſis, annis plus viginti "ſe torquet ac diſcruciat in Grammatica; "prorſus felicem ſe fore ratus, ſi tamdiu li-"ceat vivere, donec certo ſtatuat quomodo "diſtinguendæ ſint octo partes orationis, quod "hactenus nemo Græcorum aut Latinorum "ad

that grammar, as it leads only to the knowledge of words, is not deſerving of ſo much attention; for as Dr. Reid, in his very judicious account of Ariſtotle's Logic has truly obſerved, the philoſophy of grammar and that of the human underſtanding are more nearly allied than is commonly imagined. On the whole, the work in queſtion has conſiderable merit, and well deſerved the recommendation his friend Melanchton gave of it. Yet our author had no reaſon to be diſpleaſed at his other learned friend Dean Colet for not making it a ſchool book; ſince it is rather to be conſidered as a grammatical commentary for the uſe of critics, than as one of thoſe leſſer ſyſtems ſuited to young perſons at that early period of life uſually ſpent in grammar ſchools."

“ ad plenum præſtare valuit.” Linacre ſeems to have been engaged in this work by his friend Dean Colet, for the uſe of Paul’s ſchool, of which he was founder; but when it was finiſhed, the Dean preferred his own more familiar Introduction to Grammar, eſteeming this more full and accurate treatiſe on the ſubject as rather fitted for critics than learners. Linacre reſented this ſuppoſed neglect; and Eraſmus, their common friend, interpoſed to conciliate matters. The work was, however, long conſidered as a claſſic, and ſeveral editions of it were printed. The firſt came out in December 1524, a little after the death of the author.

With reſpect to Linacre’s character in his own profeſſion, as the medical writings he has left are only tranſlations, we muſt form our judgment from the great attention he paid to the ſtudy of his art, and the univerſal reputation he acquired among his countrymen and cotemporaries for ſkill in the practice of it. An inſtance of his ſagacity is recorded in a prognoſtic he made concerning his friend Lily, the celebrated grammarian, whoſe certain

tain death he foretold if he ſhould conſent to the exciſion of a malignant tumour on his hip; and the event verified his prediction. Eraſmus, in a letter to Bilibaldus Pirckheimerus, gives a very particular account of the manner in which he was relieved by the directions of Linacre in a fit of the gravel, where a ſmall ſtone ſeems to have ſtuck in the ureter: and the rational ſimplicity of the method inculcates a favourable idea of our phyſician's practice. He ſays, his friend, whoſe aſſiduity in attendance was equal to his knowledge, ſent for an apothecary to his chamber, and cauſed him in his preſence to prepare the following remedy. Camomile flowers and parſley were tied up in a linen cloth, and boiled in a veſſel of pure water till half the liquor was exhauſted; the cloth was then wrung out, and applied hot to the affected part, and eaſe was preſently procured. In a violent attack, this remedy, on the ſecond application, brought away a ſtone as big as an almond.

An Engliſh book, entitled *Compendious Regiment, or a Dietary of Health uſed at Mount-pillour*

pillour, is by ſome aſcribed to Linacre, but probably through miſtake, as there is a work of his cotemporary Andrew Borde with exactly the ſame title. Biſhop Tanner in his liſt of Linacre's works mentions *Macer's Herbal practyſyd by doctor Lynacre tranſlated out of Latin into Engliſh*. Lond. 12mo. and in the liſts given by Bale and Pits are *Epiſtolæ ad diverſos*, and *Diverſi generis Carmina*. I know not whether any of theſe are now to be met with.

I SHALL conclude this article with inſerting the epitaph written by Caius; which is both an elegant compoſition, and a judicious ſummary of the life and character of this eminent perſon.

Thomas Lynacrus, Regis *Henrici* VIII. medicus; vir & Græcé & Latiné, atque in re medica longe eruditiſſimus. Multos ætate ſua languentes, & qui jam animam deſponderant, vitæ reſtituit. Multa *Galeni* opera in Latinam linguam, mira & ſingulari facundia vertit. Egregium opus de emendata ſtructura Latini ſermonis, amicorum rogatu, paulo ante mortem

mortem edidit. Medicinæ ſtudioſis *Oxoniæ* publicas lectiones duas, *Cantabrigiæ* unam, in perpetuum ſtabilivit. In hac urbe Collegium Medicorum fieri ſua induſtria curavit, cujus & Præſidens proximus electus eſt. Fraudes doloſque miré peroſus; fidus amicis; omnibus juxta charus: aliquot annos antequam obierat Preſbyter factus; plenus annis, ex hac vita migravit, multum deſideratus, Anno Domini 1524, die 21 *Octobris.*

Vivit poſt Funera virtus.

Thomæ Lynacro clariſſimo Medico,
Johannes Caius poſuit, anno 1557.

WILLIAM BUTTE, OR BUTTS

WAS educated at Goneville hall, Cambridge, of which he became a fellow. In 1529 he was admitted a member of the college of phyſicians, in whoſe annals he is entered with the following character. "Vir "gravis;

" gravis; eximia literarum cognitione, ſingu-
" lari judicio, ſumma experientia, & prudenti
" conſilio Doctor." He was phyſician to king Henry VIII; and is immortalized by Shakeſpeare in his hiſtorical play on that monarch's reign, where he is repreſented as making the king witneſs to the ignominious treatment beſtowed on Cranmer by the lords of the council. Strype, in his life of that prelate, gives an account of this tranſaction, nearly the ſame with that of Shakeſpeare. As it is a curious piece of private hiſtory, and connected with our ſubject, I ſhall quote it.
" The next morning, according to the king's
" monition, and his own expectation, the
" council ſent for him by eight of the clock
" in the morning. And when he came to
" the council-chamber door, he was not per-
" mitted to enter into the council-chamber,
" but ſtood without among ſerving-men and
" lacquies above three quarters of an hour;
" many counſellors and others going in and
" out. The matter ſeemed ſtrange unto his
" ſecretary, who then attended upon him;
" which made him ſlip away to Dr. Butts, to
" whom he related the manner of the thing.

" Who by and by came, and kept my Lord " company. And yet e're he was called in- " to the council, Dr. Butts went to the king, " and told him that he had ſeen a ſtrange " ſight. What is that, ſaid the king? Mar- " ry, ſaid he, my lord of Canterbury is be- " come a lacquey, or a ſerving-man; for to " my knowledge, he hath ſtood among them " this hour almoſt at the council-chamber " door. Have they ſerved my Lord ſo? it " is well enough, ſaid the king; I ſhall talk " with them by and by." *Life of Cranmer*, p. 125.

From this anecdote we may imagine our phyſician to have been a friend to the reformation; and indeed this is confirmed by various other circumſtances. He firſt, as we are told by biſhop Tanner, invited that celebrated reformer Hugh Latimer to court. He alſo recommended Dr. Thirlby to Cranmer, by whoſe favour he afterwards became biſhop of Weſtminſter, and then of Norwich. Fox, the martyrologiſt, and biſhop Parkhurſt, ſpeak highly in praiſe of Dr. Butts.

STRYPE, in his life of Sir John Cheke, mentions this physician as a favourer of learning and reformation in general, and as the particular patron of Cheke, whom he assisted in his education and his introduction to the world with truly paternal kindness. In return, when he lay ill of the disorder which put an end to his life, Cheke addressed a letter to him, full of expressions of gratitude and pious condolence. It is in Latin, and is printed in Strype's work.

DR. BUTTS was knighted by Henry VIII. by the style of William Butts of Norfolk. He died November 17, 1545, and was buried in Fulham church. His portrait is in the picture of the delivery of the charter to the surgeon's company.

JOHN CHAMBRE.

THIS person is principally remarkable for being first named among the king's physicians

ſicians as a petitioner for the foundation of the college of phyſicians. He was educated in Merton College, Oxford, and became maſter of arts in 1502. He then travelled into Italy, and ſtudied phyſic at Padua, where he took a Doctor's degree; in which he was incorporated at Oxford in 1531. He was made phyſician to the king (Henry VIII.) on his return; and alſo appears, from a paſſage in an epiſtle of Linacre's to archbiſhop Warham, to have been domeſtic phyſician to that prelate. Linacre calls him "obſervantiſſimus paternitatis tuæ famulus."

He was in holy orders, and had ſeveral church preferments; among the reſt that of dean of the royal chapel and college adjoining to Weſtminſter hall, to which he built a very curious cloyſter at a large expence. He was likewiſe made Warden of Merton college in 1526, which poſt he reſigned in 1545, and died in 1549.

ANDREW BORDE, OR BOORDE.

WE have hitherto met with grave and respectable personages, who maintained the dignity of a liberal and learned profession: but the character we are now to introduce is of an extremely different cast; and the reputation he acquired among his cotemporaries must be considered as a symptom of still remaining barbarism in the manners of the times.

Andrew Borde, who styles himself in Latin *Andreas Perforatus*, was born at Pevensey in Sussex, towards the latter part of the fifteenth century. He was educated in Oxford; and before he had taken a degree, entered among the Carthusians in or near London. After some time he left them, and applied to the study of physic at Oxford; and then took a ramble through most parts of Europe, and part of Africa. On his return, he settled at Win-

Winchester, and practised in his profession with considerable reputation. In 1541 and 1542 we find him residing at Montpellier, where he probably took the degree of Doctor, in which he was soon after incorporated at Oxford. He then lived for some time at Pevensey, and afterwards returned to Winchester. Here he constantly practised the austerities of the order to which he had formerly belonged, and professed celibacy, writing with vehemence against such ecclesiastics as broke their vows by marriage. This, perhaps, was the reason why he was accused by a married bishop of violating his own pretensions to chastity by more illicit indulgencies. It is certain that his character was very odd and whimsical, as will appear more particularly from the books he wrote; yet we are told that he was esteemed in his time both as a man of great wit and learning, and an excellent physician. In this latter capacity he is said to have served king Henry VIII. As Winchester was then a royal residence, he perhaps might be his majesty's titular physician for that place. He is also mentioned as a member of the college of physicians. That he was not, however, of ſuch eminence as to rank with the firſt of his profeſſion, may be inferred from his becoming a priſoner in the Fleet, where he died in April 1549. Bale, who bore no good will to any perſon attached to popery, intimates that Borde haſtened his death by poiſon on the diſcovery of his keeping a brothel for his brother batchelors.

He was the author of ſeveral works, very various in their ſubjects. One of the moſt conſiderable of them is entitled *A Book of the Introduction of Knowledge*, profeſſing to teach all kinds of languages, the cuſtoms and faſhions of all countries, and the value of every ſpecies of coin. It is written partly in verſe and partly in proſe; and is divided into thirty-nine chapters, before each of which is a wooden cut, repreſenting a man in the habit of ſome particular country. His well-known ſatire on the Engliſhman, who to expreſs the inconſtancy and mutability of his faſhions, is drawn naked, with a piece of cloth and a pair of ſheers in his hand, is borrowed, as I am informed, from the Venetians, who characterized the French in this manner.

To

To the ſeventh chapter is prefixed the effigies of the author, under a canopy, with a gown, a laurel on his head, and a book before him. The title of the chapter declares that therein is ſhewn how the author dwelt in Scotland and *other iſlands*, and went through and round about Chriſtendom. This ſingular work was printed in London in 1542.

THE firſt of his medical works is entitled *The Breviarie of Health*. It was publiſhed in 1547; and Fuller ſuppoſes it the earlieſt medical piece written in Engliſh. It has a *prologue* addreſſed to phyſicians, which begins in this curious ſtyle. "Egregious doctors and "maſters of the eximious and arcane ſcience "of phyſick, of your urbanity exaſperate not "yourſelves againſt me for making this little "volume." The work itſelf contains a ſhort account in alphabetical order, of all diſeaſes and their remedies, adapted to the uſe of the vulgar. It is a very trifling and weak performance, extremely coarſe in language, and injudicious in matter, though perhaps not more ſo than ſome much later works of the ſame kind. The appellations of diseases in Arabic, Greek, Latin, and the barbarous medical dialect are professed to be given, but from the ignorance of the author, or blundering of the printer, the words are almost all made barbarous. That a good share of this, however, belongs to the author, appears from many strange mistakes which could only proceed from him, of which one of the most curious is his derivation of the word *Gonorrhea* from *Gomorrha*. He does not confine his attention to diseases of the body, but also treats of those of the mind; as in the following instance, which may serve for a specimen of his manner.

" *The* 174 *Chapiter doth shewe of an " infirmitie named Hereos.*

" HEREOS is the Greke worde. In Latin " it is named *Amor*. In English it is named " love sicke, and women may have this sicke-" nes as well as men. Yong persons be " much troubled with this impediment.

" *The cause of this infirmitie.*

" THIS infirmitie doth come of amours, " which is a fervent love for to have carnal copu-

" copulacion with the party that is loved; " and it cannot be obteyned ſome be ſo fool- " iſh that they be raviſhed of theyr wittes.

" *A remedy.*

" FIRST I do advertiſe every perſon not to " ſet to the hart that another doth ſet at the " hele, let no man ſet his love ſo far, but " that he may withdraw it betime, and muſe " not, but uſe mirth and mery company, and " be wyſe and not foliſh."

A MORE effectual remedy is given under the head *Satyriaſis*, for which he recommends leaping into a great veſſel of cold water, and applying nettles to the offending part.

A SECOND part of this work, containing ſome articles omitted in the firſt, is termed *the Extravagants*. They are printed together in quarto, London 1575. At the concluſion of the firſt part he ſays, " here endeth the firſt " boke, examined in Oxforde in June 1546." What is meant by this examination I cannot tell.

ANOTHER

Another medical work of this author's is entitled *Compendyous Regimente, or Dietary of Health made in Mount Pyllor*. This piece, in the edition I have of it, is printed in January 1562, ſeveral years after the author's death. It is very comprehenſive in its ſubject, containing advice concerning the ſituation and method of building a houſe, the regulating a family, and the ordering of œconomical matters, as well as directions relative to the non-naturals. There is a good deal of plain ſenſe, but very little new or ingenious in his precepts. The only part in which any thing appears worth quoting is that where he treats on the articles of diet uſual in his time.

His account of ale, which he calls natural drink for an Engliſhman, is, that it is made of malt and water, and yeſt, barme, or godsgood; and they who put any thing more to it, he ſays, ſophiſticate it. This ſhould not be drunk under five days old. Beer, he tells us, is made of malt, hops and water; and is natural drink for a Dutchman, and of late is much uſed in England to the detriment

ment of many Engliſhmen. Speaking of *wylde beaſtes' fleſhe*, he ſays; "I have gone "rounde about Chryſtendome, and over-"thwarte Chryſtendome, and a thouſand or "two and more myles oute of Chryſtendome, "yet there is not ſo muche pleaſure for Harte "and Hynde, Bucke and Doe, and for "Roobucke and Doe as is in Englande; and "although the fleſhe be diſprayſed in phyſicke "I praye God to ſende me parte of the fleſhe "to eat, phyſicke notwithſtandinge." Under the heads of roots, herbs and fruits he mentions moſt of thoſe in common uſe at this day, notwithſtanding the prevailing notion of the low ſtate of gardening among us in that period. * The title of the book, from which it would ſeem to have been drawn up at Montpellier, renders, indeed, his evidence ſomewhat doubtful; though it ſufficiently

* SIR THOMAS ELYOT in his *Caſtle of Health* enumerates the ſame. Surely Queen Katharine need not have ſent to Flanders for a ſallad, when lettuce, endive, ſuccory, beet, ſorrel and onion grew in England. It is true ſhe came over ſomewhat earlier than theſe authors wrote, but theſe articles are mentioned as quite common and of familiar uſe.

appears

appears from the contents to have been in general deſigned for the particular uſe of his countrymen. As potatoes are not at all mentioned among the articles of vegetable diet, they probably were but juſt then introduced, and not commonly known.

He is ſaid alſo to have a written a *book of Prognoſtics*, and another *of Urines*. But what is the moſt ſingular for a man of his character is his being the publiſher of a famous jeſt-book called *The Merry Tales of the Mad Men of Gotham*; and likewiſe of *The Hiſtory of the Miller of Abingdon and the Cambridge Scholars*, the ſame with that related by Chaucer in his *Canterbury Tales*. Theſe publications agree better with the biſhop's account of his conduct, than with his Carthuſian mortifications.

He left behind him in manuſcript a kind of *Tour of Europe*, deſcribing the diſtances from place to place, and the moſt remarkable objects on the road.

ABOUT

ABOUT this time flourifhed SIR THOMAS ELYOT, Knight, a perfon eminent in various branches of learning, and a patron and friend of moft of the learned men in Henry the eighth's reign. Among other works in different branches of fcience, he wrote one on phyfic, entitled *The Caftell of Health*. This was greatly efteemed, not only by the public in general, but by fome of the faculty in his time; and is, indeed, fully as worthy of notice as moft of the medical pieces of that age. Some account of it may therefore be expected in this work; though, as the author did not follow the profeffion of phyfic, he is not included in the biographical part of our plan.

THE *Caftell of Health* is faid to have been firft publifhed in 1541, yet my edition of that year is afferted to be "corrected and in fome places augmented by the firft author thereof." It was reprinted in 1572, 1580, and 1595. The writer in his *Proheme* or preface, anfwering ſwering the objection that might be raiſed againſt his work from his ſuppoſed ignorance of medical ſcience, gives an account of the manner of his acquiring this part of knowledge, which is worth quoting on account of the courſe of reading mentioned in it. "Before that I was twenty years old" he ſays, "a worſhipful Phyſician, and one of the moſt "renowned at that time in England red unto "me the works of Galen of temperaments "and natural faculties, the introduction of "Johannicius, with ſome of the Aphoriſms "of Hippocrates. And afterward by mine "own ſtudy I read over in order the more "part of the works of Hippocrates, Galen, "Oribaſius, Paulus, Celſus, Alexander, "Trallianus, Plinius the one and the other, "with Dioſcorides. Nor did I omit to read "the long canons of Avicenna, the commentaries of Averrhoes, the practiſes of "Iſaac, Haliabbas, Rhazes, Meſue; and alſo "of the more part of them which were their "aggregators and followers. And although "I have never been at Montpellier, Padua "nor Salern, yet have I found ſomething "in phyſick whereby I have taken no little "profit

" profit concerning mine own health." His acquaintaince with theſe antient authors is ſufficiently evinced in his work by his frequent references to them, and his adopting all the theory of Galen with its numerous diſtinctions and diviſions. It cannot be expected that much of original matter ſhould be found in a writer ſo circumſtanced. On the whole, his rules for diet and regimen when not drawn from Galenical theory, are founded upon good plain ſenſe; and he uniformly inculcates temperance of every kind. This he carries to a degree, with regard to certain enjoyments, that would, I preſume, be generally thought ſomewhat too rigorous, except by ſuch a bridegroom as the old gentleman in *la Fontaine*, who would be pleaſed with our knight's authority to add all the months from April to October to the red-letter days of his kalendar.

Two or three particular obſervations which appear proper to this author are all I ſhall further extract from this work. In ſpeaking of different kinds of drinks, he has the following remark concerning cyder-drinkers. "Who that " will diligently mark in the countries where " cider

" cider is uſed for a common drink, the " men and women have the colour of their " viſage pallid, and the ſkin of their viſage " rivelled, although that they be young." The qualities of the cyder of ſome counties have of late been a ſubject of much diſquiſition; and from this paſſage it will appear that ſuſpicions concerning the unwholeſomeneſs of this liquor are of long ſtanding.

FROM another paſſage we learn that the diſeaſe now called a cold began to be common in England in his time. " At this preſent time," he ſays, " in this realm of England there is not any one more annoyance " to the health of man's body, than diſtillations from the head called rheums." The cauſe of their being ſo much more frequent then than they uſed to be forty years before, he ſuppoſes to be " banquettings after ſupper, " and drinking much, ſpecially wine a little " after ſleep;" and alſo covering up the head too hot, a practice which prevailed to ſuch a degree, that he tells us " now a days if a boy of ſeven " years of age, or a young man of twenty " years have not two caps on his head, he and

" his

"his friends will think that he may not con-"tinue in health; and yet if the inner cap be "not of velvet or fattin a ferving man feareth "to lofe his credence" (credit.)

THOMAS VICARY.

THE name of this perfon deferves recording, as the author of the firft anatomical work written in the Englifh language. He was a citizen of London, Serjeant Surgeon to the kings Henry VIII. and Edward VI. and the queens Mary and Elizabeth, and chief Surgeon of St. Bartholomew's Hofpital. The title of his work is *A Treafure for Englifhmen, containing the Anatomie of Man's Body*, printed, London, 1548; or, as given by Ames, *A profitable Treatife of the Anatomy of Man's Body, compiled by* T. Vicary, *and publifhed by the Surgeons of St. Bartholomew's Hofpital*, London, 1577, 12mo. It was likewife publifhed in 1633, in 4to. together with feveral other little medical and chirurgical treatiſes. It is a ſhort piece, deſigned for the uſe of his more unlearned brethren, and taken almoſt entirely from Galen and the Arabians. A rude cut of a ſkeleton is prefixed to the latter edition.

EDWARD WOTTON

WAS born at Oxford in the year 1492, and educated at the ſchool near Magdalen College, of which college he became *Demy*, and took his batchelor's degree in 1513. Being patronized by biſhop Fox, founder of Corpus Chriſti College, and appointed *Socius Compar* and Greek lecturer of that new foundation, he continued there till 1520, when he obtained leave to travel into Italy for three years. In that country he ſtudied phyſic, and had a doctor's degree conferred on him at Padua. On his return he reſumed his lectureſhip, and was incorporated doctor of phyſic in the latter end

end of 1525. He became very eminent in his profession, first about Oxford, and then in London; and was made a member of the college of physicians in London, and physician to king Henry VIII. He died in the sixty-third year of his age, October 5th. 1555, and was buried in St. Alban's church, London. He had a son (Henry) who afterwards became an eminent physician.

Dr. Wotton appears to have been the first of our English physicians who particularly applied to a branch of study in which several have since excelled, that of Natural History. He rendered himself famous by a book on this subject, entitled *De Differentiis Animalium, lib.* X. printed, Paris 1552. Of this work the following opinion is given by the learned Gesner, in the preface to his *Historia Avium*. "Edoardus Wotton, Anglus, nuper de animalium differentiis libros decem edidit; "in quibus, etiamsi suarum observationum "quod ad historiam nihil adferat, neque novi "aliquid doceat, laude tamen & lectione "dignus est, quod pleraque veterum de animalibus scripta ita digesserit, ac inter se

" conciliarit, ut ab uno fere authore profecta " videantur omnia; stylo satis æquabili & " puro, scholiis etiam ac emendationibus uti- " lissimis adjectis, & quod priusquam ad ex- " plicandas singulorum naturas accederet, " quæ communia & in genere dici poterant, " doctissime exposuerit." This account, though drawn by a friendly hand, is not essentially different from the less favourable sentence of Haller, who says of the work, " Ab eruditione magis, quam ab ipsarum re- " rum cognitione commendatur." *Boerh. Meth. Stud. Med.*—and, " Sine ordine omnia, " fere collectitia ex veteribus, & etiam potis- " simum ex Aristotele." *Biblioth. Med.*

WOTTON also began a History of Insects, but left the finishing of it to Mouffet.

GEORGE OWEN

WAS born in the diocese of Worcester, and educated at Oxford. He became probationer fellow of Merton College in 1519, and took

took the ſeveral degrees in phyſic, that of Doctor being conferred upon him in 1527. Soon after his graduation he was made phyſician to king Henry VIII; in which office he alſo ſerved his ſucceſſors king Edward VI and queen Mary. In 1544 he was conſtituted a fellow of the College of phyſicians. His ſtation at court, and the teſtimonies of reſpectable cotemporaries, ſufficiently aſſure us of his high character in his profeſſion; but few particulars of his life important enough to be related are recorded. He was a witneſs to the will of king Henry VIII. who left him a legacy of a hundred pounds. It is reported that the ſucceeding prince, Edward VI. was brought into the world by Dr Owen's means, who performed the Cæſarian operation on his mother. From this circumſtance, whether truly or falſely related, we may conclude him to have been a practitioner in midwifery, as well as in phyſic. In the firſt year of queen Mary he was very inſtrumental in obtaining an act for the confirmation and enlargement of the powers granted to the College of Phyſicians. Some time after, in the ſame reign, upon occaſion of a difference between the College of Phyſicians and the Univerſity of Oxford, concerning the admiſſion of an illiterate perſon to a degree, who was rejected by the College upon their examination, Cardinal Pole, then Chancellor of the Univerſity, was appealed to, and obliged the Univerſity to conſult our Dr. Owen, together with Dr. Thomas Huys, the queen's phyſician, *de inſtituendis rationibus quibus Oxonienſis Academia in admittendis Medicis uteretur*. An agreement was in conſequence made, which the Chancellor approved and ratified by his authority. We learn little farther concerning this eminent phyſician, except that he enjoyed for ſeveral years before his death divers lands and tenements near Oxford, which had belonged to religious houſes, and were conferred upon him by the favour of Henry and Edward. It may from hence appear ſomewhat extraordinary, that one of his deſcendents ſhould be condemned to death in the year 1615 for maintaining the legality of killing a prince excommunicated by the Pope. Dr. Owen died October 10, 1558, of an epidemic intermittent,* and was buried in St. Stephen's, Walbrook.

LELAND

* THE account of this epidemic, as given by Dr. Caius

LELAND intimates that he had written several pieces on medical subjects, but none of them preserved. Tanner mentions the following work of his writing. *A Meet Diet for*

Caius in his annals of the College of physicians, is worth inserting.

"TERTIO die Octobris, A. D. 1558, electoi praesidis erat, quod postridie divi Michaelis ex statuto esse "nequibat; distractis hinc inde omnibus collegis in "populi subsidium; Qui febribus tertianis, duplicibus "tertianis, & tertianis continuis ita vexabatur popula- "riter per omnem mensem Augusti & Septembris, per "que universam insulam Britanniam, perinde ac peste "aliqua, ut nullus locus quieti aut privatis negotiis esse "potuit. Ex hoc morbo periere multi, non in urbe "solum, sed ruri etiam; inter quos Urbanus Huys erat, "quod dolens refero, ex immodica fatigatione per aestus "graviores, dum aulicos curaret, morbo correptus.

"PER eos menses vix erant sani, qui aegris ministra- "rent; vix messores qui messem meterent, aut in hor- "reum recolligerent. Hos morbos exceperunt quarta- "nae populariter, ut non alias aeque per hominum me- "moriam; & aliquot quintanae & octonae etiam, sed hae "breves & sine periculo: Illae plurimos de vita sustule- "runt, flores videlicet gravitatis, consilii & aetatis ma- "turae. Ex his Georgius Owenus erat, regius medicus "& Doctor Oxoniens. qui obiit" &c.

 the

the new Ague ſet forth by Mr. Dr. Owen. London 1558, fol.

ROBERT RECORDE

WAS born in Wales, and went to Oxford for his education about the year 1525. In 1531, he was elected fellow of All Soul's College. Turning his ſtudies to phyſic, but where, or under what maſters, we are not told, he was created doctor in that faculty at Cambridge in 1545. Both before and after this period he is ſaid to have taught Arithmetic at Oxford, and to have excelled all his predeceſſors in rendering this branch of knowledge clear and familiar. He is likewiſe mentioned as remarkably ſkilled in Rhetoric, Aſtronomy, Geometry, Muſic, Mineralogy, and every part of Natural Hiſtory. He was well acquainted with the Saxon language; and made large collections of hiſtorical and other

other antient manuſcripts.* To theſe various ſtudies he joined that of divinity, and was attached to the principles of the reformers. But notwithſtanding he was juſtly regarded as a prodigy of learning and parts, it does not appear that he met with encouragement at all adequate to his merits; ſince all that we know further of him is, that he died in the King's-bench priſon, where he was confined for debt, in the year 1558.

THE principal of his works are the following.

The Ground of Arts, teaching the work and practiſe of Arithmetic, both in whole numbers and Fractions. 1540. I have a republication of this in 1570, *London*, 12mo. It is dedicated to king Edward VI. In the epiſtle dedicatory, he ſays, he has omitted ſome things which were not to be publiſhed without his highneſs's approbation, " namely,

* BALE, ſpeaking of *William Batecumbe*, ſays, " In " muſæo doctoris Roberti Recorde, medici peritiſſimi, " ejus librum de ſpheræ concavæ fabrica & uſu vidi." He alſo refers to the ſame collection on other occaſions.

" becauſe

"because in them is declared all the rates "of alloyes for all ſtandards from one ounce "upward, with other myſteries of mynte "matters, and alſo moſte parte of the varie-"ties of coynes that have bin currant in this "your Majeſtie's realm by the ſpace almoſt "of ſix hundred yeares laſte paſt, and many "of them that were currant in the tyme that "the Romains ruled heere. All which, with "the aunciente deſcription of Englande and "Ireland, and my ſimple cenſure of the "ſame, I have almoſt completed to be exhi-"bited to your highneſſe." As the coin was moſt notoriouſly adulterated by the miniſtry of Edward, it is probable that this propoſed publication was not encouraged.

The Whetſtone of Wit; a ſecond part to the former.

The Path-way to Knowledge, containing the firſt principles of Geometry.

The Caſtle of Knowledge, containing the explanation of the Sphere.

The

The Urinal of Physick. This is dedicated in 1547, and was reprinted in London in 1582, 1599, and 1665. Haller, in his *Biblioth. Anat.* mentions it as containing a defcription of the urinary veffels with figures.

The Judicial of Urines. This I imagine to be the fame with the former, only with a different title; fince my edition of 1665 contains the figures and defcription that are referred to by Haller. It is a fhort, but very methodical treatife, full of divifions and fubdivifions relative to the different kinds of urines, and the prognoftics to be deduced from them. He candidly acknowledges at the beginning, that the judgment to be formed in difeafes from the urine is not fo certain as fome have reprefented; and indeed the perplexity and variety of opinions concerning this fubject are fufficiently apparent from his treatife.

Of Anatomy.
Of Auricular Confeffion.
Of the Euchariſt.
The Image of a True Commonwealth.

ALBAYN

ALBAYN HYLL

WAS born in Wales, or, according to Dempſter, in Scotland, and educated partly at Oxford, and partly in a foreign univerſity, where he applied to the ſtudy of phyſic, and took a Doctor's degree. He was famous for his practice in London, and was much admired by his learned cotemporaries both in England and abroad. He had a particular intimacy with the learned Dr. Caius and Dr. Fryer of Cambridge. It is probable he lived a good deal in foreign countries, ſince the chief accounts we have of him come from foreigners. Joſias Simler of Zurick, and Baſſianus Landus of Placentia mention him with honour: the latter ſtyles him "medicus nobiliſſimus atque optimus, & in omni literarum genere maxime verſatus;" and tells us that he wrote ſeveral pieces upon Galen, particularly the anatomical part of his works. He

He died December 26, 1559, and was buried in St. Alban's church, London.

FULLER mentions it as ſomewhat remarkable, that Wales had three eminent phyſicians and writers who were cotemporaries; viz. Recorde, Phayer, and Hyll.

THOMAS PHAYER OR PHAIRE

WAS born in Pembrokeſhire, and educated at Oxford, from whence he removed to Lincoln's Inn for the ſtudy of the law. This he purſued to ſuch length as to become an author in it, writing a treatiſe on the nature of Writs, and another of the ſame kind with that now called a book of Precedents. For ſome reaſon, however, with which we are not acquainted, he quitted the law, and with equal ardour purſued the ſtudy of phyſic. He took his degree of Doctor in this faculty at Oxford in 1559; but ſo long before as the year

year 1544 we find him publiſhing a tranſlation of a French treatiſe concerning *the Peſtilence*, together with *a Deſcription of the Veins in the Human Body*, and the purpoſes anſwered by opening each of them. From the ſame language he alſo tranſlated a book on *the Diſeaſes of Children*, one of *Regimen*, and one of *Remedies, or Medical Preſcriptions*. This is the account given of his medical works; but in the preface to a collection of them in my poſſeſſion, printed, *London* 1560, he only acknowledges the *Regiment of Life* to be a tranſlation from the French, but it is ſaid of the *Treatiſe on the Peſtilence*, and the *Boke of Children* that they are "compoſed by Thomas "Phayer, ſtudious in philoſophie and "phiſycke." They are however mere compilations, with little or nothing of his own. He ſeems to have been in conſiderable reputation for his medical practice, but where he exerciſed it is not ſo clear. Bale ſays he flouriſhed at London in 1550; Pits, that he died there in that year; but Wood, who appears to be better informed, traces his reſidence in South Wales from the year 1555 to 1560, when he died at Kilgarran in Pembrokeſhire;

brokeſhire; in which place he was alſo buried.

Among his various attainments, his poetical abilities were not the leaſt famous in his time. He wrote in verſe *An account of Owen Glendour, who deceived by falſe prophecies aſſumed the title of Prince of Wales*; and likewiſe undertook a *Tranſlation of the Æneid*, which ſeems to have been the great employment of the latter part of his life, but of which he only finiſhed nine books. Pits characterizes this performance as being done "magna gravitate, pari elegantia:" but Fuller ſays, the wits of his time would render this *gravitas* "dullneſs;" and deſcribes the verſification as extremely rude and inharmonious.

WILLIAM TURNER.

We have already ſeen that ſome of the phyſicians of this period paid a particular

cular attention to the ſtudy of natural hiſtory. The circumſtances of the times, in which the principles of reformation in religion were every where ſtruggling againſt an antient and powerful eſtabliſhment, gave alſo a turn towards theological enquiries to almoſt all who were habituated to ſtudy and ſpeculation; among whom thoſe of the medical profeſſion were always conſpicuous. A threefold union of the ſeveral characters of phyſician, naturaliſt, and divine was therefore not unfrequent at this æra; and there were few in whom it exiſted more eminently than in the ſubject of the following memoirs.

William Turner was born at Morpeth in Northumberland. He was educated at Cambridge, where, as we find from a dedicatory epiſtle of his to Lord Wentworth, he was aſſiſted by a yearly exhibition from that nobleman's father. In this univerſity he purſued the ſtudies of philoſophy and phyſic; and alſo acquired a great reputation for proficiency in the learned languages, oratory and poetry. He was a fellow-collegian and friend of the celebrated biſhop Ridley, and imbibed, together

together with him, the religious principles of the reformers, which then began to be received in England. In his zeal for the propagation of theſe opinions, he for ſome time quitted his medical purſuits, and tratravelled through the greateſt part of the kingdom as an itinerant and unlicenſed preacher.* For this, at the inſtigation of biſhop Gardiner and others, he was impriſoned; and on his eſcape, or, as Wood repreſents it, his releaſe, he baniſhed himſelf to foreign

* As a ſpecimen of the ſtyle of the Oxford antiquary, Anthony Wood, and his manner of treating an *innovator* and oppoſer of an *eſtabliſhment*, though that eſtabliſhment was popery, I ſhall quote his repreſentation of this matter. "This perſon, (Turner) who was very conceited "of his own worth, hot headed, a buſy body, and "much addicted to the opinions of Luther, would needs "in the heighth of his ſtudy of phyſic turn Theologiſt, "but always refuſed the uſual ceremonies to be obſerved "in order to his being made Prieſt: and whether he had "orders conferred upon him according to the R. Cath. "manner, appears not. Sure it is, that while he was a "young man, he went unſent for, through many parts "of the nation, and preached the word of God, not "only in towns and villages, but alſo in cities." *Athen. Oxon*, II. 154.

countries. He took the degree of doctor of physic at Ferrara; and during the remainder of Henry the eighth's reign he resided chiefly at Cologne and other places in Germany, where he published some of his works. In the next reign, which was more agreeable to his religious opinions, he returned to England, and was very favourably received by the young king, who presented him with a prebend of York, a canonry of Windsor, and the deanery of Wells. He likewise obtained a license to read and preach, as many other learned laymen did at that time; and was incorporated doctor of physic at Oxford. The protector, Edward, duke of Somerset, made him his physician; which brought him into considerable practice among people of rank. On the accession of queen Mary he was again obliged to quit his country, and went into Germany with several other English divines; from thence to Rome, and afterwards for a time settled in Basil. At her death he returned, and was restored to his preferments. He died July 7th. 1568, and was buried in St. Olave's church yard, London.

HE

He left a widow, who afterwards married Dr. Richard Cox, biſhop of Ely; and ſeveral children, one of whom was a doctor of phyſic, whoſe ſon was Geometry profeſſor in Greſham College.

Dr. Turner was a writer in all the three branches of knowledge for which he was eminent. His medical works are

A book of the nature and properties of Bathes in England, as of other Bathes in Germany and Italy. Colen, 1562. fol. A preface to this, addreſſed "to his well beloved neighbours in Bath, Briſtol, Wells, Wynſam, and Charde" is dated from Baſil, March 10. 1557. In it he ſays, that as far as he can learn, he is the firſt writer on the waters of Bath. A dedication of the work to the earl of Hertford is dated, London, Feb. 15, 1560. His account of foreign baths is ſhort and chiefly taken from other authors. That of the Engliſh is confined to thoſe of Bath. Theſe he ſuppoſes to be impregnated with no other mineral than ſulphur. He complains much of the little care taken of them, and the want of conveniences to render them proper for the ſick. He propoſes ſome alterations, and recommends the refuſe water to be collected for the purpoſe of bathing diſeaſed horſes. He mentions nothing of their internal uſe.

The nature of Wines commonly uſed in England, with a confutation of them that hold that Rheniſh and other ſmall wines ought not to be drunken, either of them that have the ſtone, the rheum, or other diſeaſes. London 1568, 8vo. With this was printed a *Treatiſe on the nature and vertue of Triacle.*

The rare treaſure of Engliſh Bathes. London, 1587, 4to. I have a piece with this title and author's name, printed with ſome other old medical tracts, which is ſaid to be "gathered "and ſet forth for the benefit of the poorer "ſort of people by William Bremer practiti-"oner in phyſic and chirurgerie." It relates only to the bath of Bath, and chiefly conſiſts of directions for its uſe.

Dr. Turner was author of the firſt *Herbal* written

written in the Engliſh language. The firſt part of this Herbal was printed in London in 1551; A ſecond part, addreſſed to lord Wentworth, at Colen, 1562. They are both in folio; and wooden cuts, many of them not inelegant, are prefixed to the account of each plant. The author mentions that botanical ſtudies were ſo much neglected in England, that, about the middle of Henry the eighth's reign, he found not a ſingle phyſician at Cambridge who could inform him of the Greek, Latin, or Engliſh name of any plant he produced.

In Natural Hiſtory he likewiſe publiſhed a ſmall treatiſe on birds, entitled

Avium præcipuarum, quarum apud Plinium & Ariſtotelem mentio eſt, brevis & ſuccincta hiſtoria. Colon. 1554, 12mo. It is written in elegant Latin, and is a book, as Dr. Merret obſerves, "mole parvum, judicio majorem." He was cotemporary with Geſner, and a correſpondent in high eſteem with that illuſtrious naturaliſt. In the Frankfort edition of Geſner's *Hiſtoria Piſcium* is a letter of our countryman's to him, giving a ſhort account of the Britiſh fiſh, alſo their Engliſh names. This letter is dated at Weiſſenberg, November 1557, where Turner practiſed phyſic; Geſner calling him "Medicus Weiſſenburgi eximius." He again, in the preface to his ornithology, ſpeaks very reſpectfully of our countryman's knowledge of that ſubject, and ſeldom omits quoting him whenever he has opportunity.*

The religious writings of our author were numerous, and many of them had the quaint and affected titles uſual in thoſe days. Strype, in his *Life of Cranmer*, p. 357 gives the following account of one of them, which I ſhall quote as a ſpecimen of his manner. It is entitled, *A New Book of Spiritual Phyſick for divers diſeaſes of the Nobility and Gentlemen of England*; printed 1555, and dedicated to ſeveral of the principal nobility. "It conſiſt-"ed of three parts. In the firſt he ſhewed "who were noble and gentlemen, and how "many works and properties belong unto

* For the above paragraph I am indebted to Mr. Pennant.

"ſuch,

" ſuch, and wherein their office chiefly ſtand-
" eth. In the ſecond part he ſhewed great
" diſeaſes were in the Nobility and Gentry,
" which letted them from doing their office.
" In the third part he ſpecified what the diſ-
" eaſes were: as namely, the whole palſy, the
" dropſy, the Romiſh pox, and the leproſy;
" ſhewing afterwards the remedies againſt
" theſe diſeaſes. For being a very facetious
" man, he delivered his reproofs and counſels
" under witty and pleaſant diſcourſe."

THOMAS GIBSON

WAS a townſman and a cotemporary of Turner, and like him united divinity and natural hiſtory with medicine. He was alſo eminent for hiſtorical knowledge. He probably ſtudied at Oxford, but at what preciſe time we are not acquainted. To his character as a phyſician Bale bears witneſs, by ſaying that he performed moſt incredible cures. He was a friend to the reformation, and wrote ſeveral pieces for the ſervice of that cauſe. In the reign of queen Mary he was a fugitive for his religion, but on the acceſſion of Elizabeth returned, and died at London in 1562. Tanner gives the following liſt of his writings.

A Breve Chronicle of the biſhops of Rome's bleſſynge, and of his prelates beneficial and charitable rewards, from the tyme of king Heralde to this daye (in Engliſh rhyme) London 12mo. This, I ſuppoſe, is the work called by others *The treaſons of the prelates.*

The Sum of the Acts and Decrees made by divers biſhops of Rome. Tranſlated from the Latin. 12mo.

Of the Ceremonies uſed by Popes.

A Treatiſe behooveful as well to preſerve the people from Peſtilence, as to help and recover them that be infected with the ſame, made by a Biſhop and Dr. of Phyſic in Denmark, which Medicines

Medicines have been proved in many places in London. 1536, 4to.

An Herbal.

Treatiſe againſt unſkilful Alchimiſts.

Treatiſe of curing common Diſeaſes.

De utroque homine, lib. I.

The various States that Britany hath been in (ſuppoſed to be left imperfect.)

ONE of his name, ſuppoſed by Wood to be himſelf, made application of ſome paſſages in the prophetic writings to the circumſtances of his own time, in favour of king Henry VIII. —a deluſion too common among the proteſtants of that age.

JOHN CLEMENT.

AT what preciſe time, or in what part of England this learned phyſician was born, we are not informed. He was educated at Oxford, and was honoured with a very early

early acquaintance with Sir Thomas More, who took him into his family, made him tutor to his children, and seems to have regarded him with paternal kindness. The following passage in a letter from that illustrious person to Petrus Ægidius*, is a pleasing declaration of his sentiments concerning Clement, and his treatment of him. He is speaking of a literary difficulty started by his young friend. "Nam et Joannes Clemens "puer meus, qui adfuit, ut scis, una, ut "quem a nullo patior sermone abesse, in quo "aliquid esse fructus potest, quoniam ab hac "herba, quæ et Latinis literis & Græcis cæ-"pit evirescere, egregiam aliquando frugem "spero, in magnam me conjecit dubitatio-"nem." In another letter he mentions him as teaching Greek to Colet, afterwards Dean of St. Paul's, and founder of Paul's school.

The friendship of Sir Thomas More was not of such an interested nature, as to be a restraint upon the advancement of Clement. On the contrary, we find him, about the year

* Jortin's Erasmus, Vol. II. p. 625.

1519,

1519, ſettled at Corpus Chriſti College in Oxford, as profeſſor of rhetoric, and afterwards of Greek, in that Univerſity, in conſequence of his patron's recommendation to Cardinal Wolſey. Theſe employments he filled with great reputation; and it is remarked, to the honour of the medical faculty, that as Linacre was the firſt who taught Greek at Oxford, ſo Clement was the ſecond teacher there of any note in that language. Till this period it does not appear that his ſtudies had been directed to any particular profeſſion; but he now gave himſelf up entirely to the purſuit of medical knowledge. Thus More, in one of his epiſtles, mentioning Lupſet as profeſſor of the languages at Oxford, ſays, "Succeſſit enim Joanni Cle-"menti meo; nam is ſe totum addixit rei "Medicæ, nemini aliquando ceſſurus, niſi "hominem (quod abominor) hominibus in-"inviderint Parcæ." * This was in the year 1520 or 1521. His ſucceſs in medical ſtudies appears to have been ſuch as might have been expected from his learning and abilities.

* Jortin *ibid.* Vol. II. p. 396.

He

He was made a Fellow of the College of Phyſicians in London; and was one of the phyſicians ſent by Henry VIII. to Wolſey, when he lay languiſhing at Eſher in 1529. In the reign of Edward VI. he left his country for the ſake of the Roman Catholic religion, a ſtrong attachment to which he had probably imbibed in the family of his patron Sir Thomas More. Some circumſtances muſt have rendered him peculiarly obnoxious to the court, ſince we find him, with ſome other papiſts, excepted from a general pardon granted by Edward in the year 1552. It was during his continuance abroad on this occaſion, that, as Wood thinks, he took the degree of doctor of phyſic. On the acceſſion of Queen Mary he returned, and practiſed in his profeſſion in a part of Eſſex, near London. At her death he went abroad a ſecond time, and there ſpent the remainder of his days. He died at Mechlin, where he had reſided and practiſed ſeveral years, on July 1ſt. 1572.

He married, about the year 1526, a lady named Margaret, who was in the family of Sir

Sir Thomas More at the ſame time with himſelf. Pits calls her "Margaritam illam, "quam inter filias ſuas, tanquam filiam, "educari fecerat Morus." She was little inferior to her huſband in knowledge of the learned languages, and gave him conſiderable aſſiſtance in his tranſlations from the Greek. She lived with him above forty-four years, dying in 1570; and in an epitaph which he wrote for her monument, among other ſubjects of praiſe, he relates her teaching her ſons and daughters Greek and Latin.

The only works which Clement publiſhed were ſome tranſlations of pieces in divinity from the Greek, and a book of Latin epigrams and other verſes.

THOMAS GALE.

FROM the writings of this author the following circumſtances of his life are collected.

He

He was born in 1507; and educated under Richard Ferris, afterwards Serjeant Surgeon to queen Elizabeth. He was a ſurgeon in the army of king Henry VIII. at Montruil, in 1544; and alſo in that of king Philip at St. Quintin, in 1557. He afterwards ſettled in London, and became very eminent in the practice of ſurgery. He was living in 1586. Biſhop Tanner gives the following liſt of his writings.

The Inſtitution of a Chirurgeon. An Enchiridion of Surgery, in four books. *On Gunſhot Wounds. Antidotary*, two books. All theſe were printed together, *London*, 1563, 8vo.

A Compendious Method of curing Præternatural Tumours. On the ſeveral kinds of Ulcers and their cure. A Commentary on Guido de Cauliaco. Theſe are mentioned by W. Cunningham in his prefatory epiſtle to the Inſtitution of a Chirurgeon.

An Herbal for the uſe of Surgeons. This he promiſes towards the end of his Enchiridion.

A Brief

A Brief Declaration of the Art of Medicine, and the Office of a Chirurgeon. An Epitome of Galen de natural. facultat. Theſe two are printed with a tranſlation of *Galen de Methodo Medendi.*

THE *Inſtitution of a Chirurgeon,* and the other works printed with it, are dedicated to Lord Robert Dudley, Maſter of the Horſe to the queen (Elizabeth). The date is July 16, 1563.

THE *Inſtitution* is a dialogue in which Gale, and John Field, another ſurgeon who was educated with him under Ferris, are repreſented as anſwering the queſtions of a ſtudent, John Yates. It is a general Introduction to Surgery, containing a definition of the art, with its ſeveral branches; a brief account of the inſtruments and apparatus uſed in it; definitions of all the diſeaſes in which it is converſant; tables of the different kinds of wounds, ulcers, fractures, diſlocations, &c.; and a deſcription of ligatures, ſutures, tents and dreſſings.

The *Enchiridion* is a plain and concise account of the method of practice in curing wounds, fractures, and dislocations. It is extracted from former writers in surgery, and contains nothing of his own except a powder for stopping the hæmorrhage after amputation, without the cautery. This, he says, "was "invented by himself and one master Pier-"ponte, and first put in use and practice by "the surgeons in St. Thomas's hospital in "Southwarke. And since that time put in "use of many more, both young and old, "not onely in taking off members, but re-"straining of blood both in veins and arteries, "which could not be done with hot irons." He further declares that he has not known two die on whom this powder was used after amputating the leg or arm. The recipe is as follows. R. *Aluminis succarini, Thuris, Arsenici aa* ℥ij *Calcis vivi* ℥vi. Powder them together, and boil them in a pint of strong vinegar to the consumption of the liquor. Take of the dry residuum three ounces, *Bole Armoniack* half an ounce, *Pulvis Alcamisticus* one ounce. Reduce them to a very fine powder, and you have the medicine required. The method of using

uſing it is to mix it with white of egg, and ſpread it upon tow, ſprinkling upon it ſome of the dry powder; and apply over the end of the ſtump.

His *Treatiſe on Gun-ſhot Wounds*, is chiefly deſigned to confute the error of Jerome of Brunſwick, John de Vigo, Alphonſus Ferrius and others, in ſuppoſing theſe wounds to be of a venomous nature; an error of bad conſequence in practice. Our author quotes the opinions of Galen and Dioſcorides concerning the ingredients of which gun-powder is made, ſhewing from thence that they were uſed as medicines inſtead of being conſidered as poiſonous. It is, however, to be obſerved, that he miſtakes the nitre of the antients for ſaltpetre. He alſo proves that the bullet does not acquire ſuch a heat in its motion as to render its wound ſimilar to a cautery, which was the common opinion. From hence he adopts a milder method of treating theſe wounds, directing his endeavours to the procuring a laudable digeſtion, and in all reſpects conſidering them as common contuſions. Some of his remedies, however, are ſharper than modern practice allows in these cases; such as ointments with *precipitate* and *ægyptiacum*. In our account of William Clowes, a nearer approach to the best modern practice, introduced by that surgeon, will be remarked. Some short chapters, in which the variations of treatment in gun-shot wounds, according to the different parts they occupy, are mentioned, compose the rest of this treatise.

The *Antidotarie* is a collection of chirurgical receipts, mostly extracted from other authors, but some of his own invention. Among the rest, are a few of Sir William Butts's, particularly two of plasters directed by that physician for king Henry VIII. when troubled with swelled legs. None of these *formulæ*, however, deserve attention at present.

Another volume of this surgeon's works is dated in 1566, and dedicated to Sir Henry Neville. The two first pieces contained in it are entitled *A brief Declaration of the worthy Art of Medicine*, and the *Office of a Chirurgion*. The chief purport of these tracts is to give a general history of the healing art, and to inculcate

culcate a proper idea of the neceſſity of a ſcientific method of ſtudy in attaining it, and of the connexion between its ſeveral branches. Numerous complaints of the intruſion of illiterate pretenders and empiricks into the practice of medicine and ſurgery are interſperſed through theſe pieces; ſome of which are worth notice, as containing curious information of the ſtate of the profeſſion at that time. The deplorable condition of military practice may be judged from the following relation. "I remember," ſays he, "when I "was in the wars, at Muttrel, in the time of "that moſt famous prince king Henry VIII. "there was a great rabblement there, that "took upon them to be ſurgeons. Some "were ſow-gelders, and ſome horſe-gelders, "with tinkers and coblers. This noble ſect "did ſuch great cures, that they got them-"ſelves a perpetual name; for like as Theſ-"ſalus' ſect were called Theſſalions, ſo was "this noble rabblement, for their notorious "cures, called dog-leaches; for in two dreſ-"ſings they did commonly make their cures "whole and ſound for ever, ſo that they nei-"ther felt heat nor cold, nor no manner of

" pain after. But when the duke of Norfolk, " who was then general, underſtood how the " people did die, and that of ſmall wounds, " he ſent for me, and certain other ſurgeons, " commanding us to make ſearch how theſe " men came to their death, whether it were " by the grievouſneſs of their wounds, or by " the lack of knowledge of the ſurgeons; and " we according to our commandment made " ſearch through all the camp, and found ma-" ny of the ſame good fellows, which took " upon them the names of ſurgeons, not only " the names, but the wages alſo. We aſking " of them whether they were ſurgeons, or no, " they ſaid they were; we demanded with " whom they were brought up, and they, with " ſhameleſs faces, would anſwer, either with " one cunning man, or another, which was " dead. Then we demanded of them what " chirurgery ſtuff they had to cure men with-" all; and they would ſhew us a pot, or a " box, which they had in a budget, wherein " was ſuch trumpery as they did uſe to greaſe " horſes heels withall, and laid upon ſcabbed " horſes backs, with nerval, and ſuch like. " And other, that were coblers and tinkers,

" they

"they used shoe-maker's wax, with the rust "of old pans, and made therewithall a noble "salve, as they did term it. But in the end, "this worthy rabblement was committed to "the Marshalsea, and threatened by the duke's "grace to be hanged for their worthy deeds, "except they would declare the truth what "they were, and of what occupations, and in "the end they did confess, as I have declared "to you before."

At this period, however, as we are informed in a subsequent paragraph, the number of regular bred surgeons to supply the public service was much greater than afterwards. For when he is lamenting the wretched state of the profession, he says, "I have, myself, "in the time of king Henry VIII. holpe to "furnish out of London in one year which "served by sea and land, threescore and "twelve surgeons, which were good work-"men, and well able to serve, and all En-"glishmen. At this present day there are "not thirty-four of all the whole company of "Englishmen, and yet the most part of them "be in noblemen's service, so that, if we

" ſhould have need, I do not know where to " find twelve ſufficient men. What do I ſay? " ſufficient men: nay I would there were ten " amongſt all the company, worthy to be " called ſurgeons."

Our author, in his *Office of a Chirurgeon*, takes notice of a report raiſed in order to injure him, that Dr. Cuningham, and not himſelf, was the writer of the works formerly publiſhed by him. He acknowledges that " not having perfect underſtanding of the " tongues, he required him, for the more " perfection thereof, to put in the Greek and " Latin words, in ſuch ſort as he thought " good;" but contends that the matter was his own, and the caſes related derived from his own practice.*

The reſt of this volume conſiſts of tranſlations, of the 3d, 4th, 5th, and 6th books of Galen's *Therapeuticon*; of his book *on præter-*

* In the preface to the former volume, he mentions that Dr. Cuningham " was no ſmall help to him in " deviſing the arguments, and peruſing the copies " written."

natural

natural tumours, and an epitome of his three books *of natural faculties*. How far his friend Cuningham was aſſiſting in theſe, we are not told; but from the confeſſion above-mentioned it is reaſonable to ſuppoſe that he would be applied to on the occaſion.

JOHN KAYE OR KEY,

MORE generally known by the name of CAIUS, may be regarded as the ſucceſſor of Linacre in uniting the firſt honours of literature with thoſe of medicine.

HE was born at Norwich, October 6, 1510; and after receiving the firſt rudiments of learning in that city, he was ſent very young to Cambridge, and admitted in Goneville Hall, of which he became fellow. His great attachment to his ſtudies was manifeſted by ſome very early productions; for, at the age of twenty-one, in order to gratify ſome of his friends, and put his abilities to the proof, he

 tranſlated

tranſlated a treatiſe of Nicephorus Calliſtus, and another of Chryſoſtom, out of Greek into Latin; and epitomized Eraſmus's book *De Vera Theologia*; and likewiſe tranſlated from Latin into Engliſh that author's paraphraſe on Jude. About ſix years after this, he loſt his intimate friend and townſman William Frammingham, of whom he gives a moſt extraordinary character for abilities and learning. This perſon left behind him eight treatiſes on various ſubjects, which he committed to the care of our young ſtudent, who ſpent much pains in writing notes and commentaries upon them.

It was probably ſoon after this that, according to the cuſtom of the times, he travelled into Italy for further improvement in thoſe branches of ſcience which he deſigned more particularly to purſue. He ſtudied phyſic at Padua under Joh. Baptiſta Montanus, the moſt eminent medical profeſſor of his time. In this city he lodged in the ſame houſe with the celebrated anatomiſt Andreas Veſalius; and ſeems to have followed anatomical ſtudies with an ardour equal to that of his

his companion. He took the degree of doctor first at Bologna. In 1542, in conjunction with Realdus Columbus, he gave public lectures on the Greek text of Aristotle, at Padua, a salary for which purpose was paid by some noble Venetians — an illustrious proof of his high character in the very seat of learning. In 1543 he made the tour of the greatest part of Italy, visiting all the most celebrated libraries, and collating manuscripts, principally with a view to the giving correct editions of the works of Galen and Celsus. At Pisa he heard the medical lectures of Mattheus Curtius; and he finished his travels with France and Germany.

On his return to his own country, he was incorporated doctor of physic at Cambridge, and practised in his profession at Shrewsbury and Norwich, with a success so favourable to his reputation, that he was called to court, and appointed physician to king Edward VI; in which capacity he afterwards served the queens Mary and Elizabeth. The precise year in which he came to the metropolis is not ascertained; but he mentions certain anatomical

tomical demonstrations which he annually exhibited before the corporation of surgeons, at the request of king Henry VIII; whence it would appear that he was settled in London during the reign of that prince.

In 1547 he was constituted a fellow of the College of Physicians; and ever after was the great ornament and support of that body, passing through all its honours, and for seven years presiding at its head. His zealous attachment to the dignity and interests of this society was manifested on various occasions. He invented those honorary *insignia* by which the president has ever since been distinguished. He was a strenuous assertor of the rights and privileges of the College, which he defended publicly, with success, in the reign of Elizabeth, against the surgeons, who claimed a right of prescribing internal medicines in certain cases where their manual assistance was requisite. His zeal was exerted, perhaps more beneficially for the public, in erecting a monument to the memory of his great predecessor, Linacre; in obtaining a grant for the College to take annually the bodies of two condemned

condemned malefactors for diſſection, the expence attending which he left a fund to defray; and in compiling the annals of that learned ſociety, from its inſtitution to the concluding year of his preſidency. He was ſo religious an obſerver of the College ſtatutes, that, even in his old age, he would not aſſume the liberty of abſenting himſelf from its aſſemblies without a particular diſpenſation.

His munificent patronage of learning in general, and grateful return to the ſociety from which he had received his education, were exemplified in a manner that does him peculiar honour. In the reign of queen Mary, with whom he was much in favour, he obtained licence to advance Goneville Hall into a College; which permiſſion he ſuitably ſeconded by endowing it with ſeveral eſtates for the maintenance of three fellows and twenty ſcholars, and by various other acts of bounty. This was effected in the courſe of the years 1557 and 1558; and his name, together with that of the co-founder, Goneville, ſtill gives title to the college. He framed a new body of laws for this ſocie-

ty,

ty, and in 1559 accepted the maſterſhip of it, which he retained as long as he lived. In 1565 he began to enlarge his College by the erection of a new ſquare; and reſigned his poſt as preſident of the College of Phyſicians, that he might the more aſſiduouſly ſuperintend this work: which was finiſhed in 1570, at the expence of one thouſand eight hundred and thirty-four pounds,—a very conſiderable ſum at that time. This capital benefaction, conferred *during his life*, and at a period of it when the paſſion for accumulating wealth is uſually ſtrongeſt, muſt be admitted as an undeniable proof both of his warm attachment to the intereſts of literature, and of his liberal and philoſophical diſpoſition.

The moralizing turn of the man, or of the age, was ſhewn by the inſcriptions he cauſed to be put over the gates of his new ſquare. One, being low and little, was inſcribed *Humilitatis*; the next, which was a portico of handſome architecture, was inſcribed *Virtutis*, and on the oppoſite ſide was written *Jo. Caius poſuit Sapientiæ*. That leading to the public ſchools, through which all paſſed for their degrees

degrees, was inſcribed *Honoris*. The good man ſeems to have derived great ſatisfaction from this diſpoſition of his bounty; for he made this manſion of learning the retreat of his old age; and after reſigning the maſterſhip, he reſided as a fellow-commoner, aſſiſting at daily prayers in the chapel, in a private ſeat built for his own uſe.

Religious diſputes ran ſo high at this period, that it was not likely, with all his generoſity and beneficence, he ſhould eſcape the effects of party rancour. In 1565 three fellows of his college whom he had expelled preferred articles againſt him, charging him not only with "ſhew of a perverſe ſtomach "to the profeſſors of the goſpel, but atheiſm." Strype obſerves upon this, that he might poſſibly affect an indifference for all religion, in order to cover his ſecret attachment to popery; the reality of which he infers from a quantity of veſtments, and other implements of public worſhip after the popiſh ceremonial, being found in his lodgings upon a ſearch, which were without mercy committed to the flames. Pits, on the other hand, a bigotted

Roman

Roman Catholic writer, accuses him of great unsteadiness and mutability in his religious principles. That he was of a compliant disposition in these matters, is evident, from his maintaining the post he occupied at court under princes of such opposite sentiments; yet it is not improbable that he had a predilection for the antient establishment. Fuller apologizes for him in a very pleasing strain of candour. His being a reputed papist, he says, "was no great crime to such who consider "the time when he was born, and foreign "places wherein he was bred. However, this "I dare say in his just defence; he never mentioneth protestants but with due respect, "and sometimes doth occasionally condemn "the superstitious credulity of popish miracles. Besides, after he had resigned his "mastership to Dr. Legge, he was constantly "present at protestant prayers. If any say, "all this amounts but to a lukewarm religion, we leave the heat of his faith to God's "sole judgment, and the light of his good "works to men's imitation." *Hist. Univ. Cambr.*

THAT

THAT our learned phyſician's retirement from the public buſineſs of his profeſſion was not owing to a fit of gloomy diſtaſte to the world, or monkiſh ſuperſtition, but a truly philoſophic fondneſs for learned leiſure, appears from the numerous pieces upon literary ſubjects which afterwards came from his pen, and in which he was engaged to the laſt period of his life. He appears to have been reduced to a ſtate of great bodily weakneſs before his death; and from a curious paſſage in Dr. Mouffet's *Health's Improvement*, or *Rules concerning Food*, we learn that he attempted to ſuſtain his decaying frame by reverting to the food of infancy. It is this. "What made Dr. Caius in his laſt ſickneſs ſo "peeviſh and ſo full of frets at Cambridge, "when he ſucked one woman (whom I ſpare "to name) froward of conditions and of bad "diet; and contrariwiſe ſo quiet and well "when he ſucked another of contrary diſ- "poſitions? verily the diverſity of their milks "and conditions, which being contrary one "to the other, wrought alſo in him that "ſucked them contrary effects." There are not

not wanting other inſtances of the ſame regimen in valetudinarians.

He died, after having foretold his death, on July 29, 1573, in the ſixty-third year of his age. He was buried within the chapel of his own college, in a grave made ſome time before his deceaſe; and by way of epitaph the following laconic inſcription was put upon his tomb—Fui Caius.

From the preceding ſummary of the life of this celebrated perſon, it will appear that he was altogether a literary character; and we are furniſhed with ample materials for conſidering him in this light, not only from the numerous works of his ſtill extant, but, in particular, from a treatiſe he drew up, in imitation of Galen, *concerning his own writings*. By this we are enabled not only to fix the date of all his productions, but to aſcertain ſeveral other circumſtances relative to them, which we are generally obliged, with regard to other authors, to ſupply by conjecture. It were to be wiſhed that other eminent and voluminous writers would pay an equal re-

gard

gard to the information of posterity. The great variety of the writings of Caius renders it necessary to distribute them into classes; and we shall separately consider those in which he appears as a critic and linguist, a physician, a naturalist, and an antiquary.

His accurate knowledge of the Greek and Latin languages, and his critical abilities, are amply evinced by his translations, his annotations, and the multitude of books of which he gave corrected editions. It has already been mentioned that his first essay in literature was the translation of certain devotional pieces from the Greek; and that he next employed himself in writing annotations on the posthumous Latin works of his friend Frammingham. These, together with the works themselves, were irrecoverably lost by those to whose hands they were entrusted during our author's absence in Italy.

While he resided in that country he wrote commentaries upon Galen's nine books *De Administrationibus Anatomicis*, and his two books *De Motu Musculorum*. These he printed after

 his

his return, together with a corrected edition of the originals, and of ſeveral other pieces of the ſame author, at the Frobenian preſs in Baſil, in the year 1544. Indeed, the correction and elucidation of the works of this great phyſician ſeemed to be an object of all others the moſt intereſting to him; and to this end he employed incredible labour in collating manuſcripts and comparing parallel paſſages: and his induſtry and ſagacity were attended with ſuch ſucceſs, that he not only gave much more correct editions of many of his pieces than had before appeared, but recovered ſome that were quite loſt in obſcurity and neglect.

The ſame ſervices he rendered in ſome degree to the great Father of phyſic, particularly by reſtoring his treatiſe *De Anatomia*, the ſubſtance of which had been concealed under another title; and that *De Medicamentis*, never before printed. It is obvious that the moſt profound and critical knowledge of the Greek language was requiſite in the execution of theſe attempts; and it is probable that no no ſcholar in Europe was at that time ſuperior, or perhaps equal to him, in that reſpect.

Nor were the early Latin medical writers leſs obliged to his critical labours. Celſus was the companion of his tour through the principal cities of Italy; and by a collation of ſeveral printed copies with the manuſcripts at Florence and Urbino, he was enabled to make large emendations of that author, as well as of his cotemporary, Scribonius Largus. Theſe he enriched with annotations; but it does not appear that they were ever committed to the preſs. At leaſt, he mentions them as lying by him in manuſcript two or three years before his death.

Under the head of his critical productions we muſt likewiſe rank a ſmall treatiſe entitled *De Symphonia Vocum Britannicarum*, in which he attempted to ſhew the conſonance of the Engliſh language with the Greek and Latin. This work, which was never publiſhed, we may ſuppoſe to have exhibited more claſſical learning than ſagacity and juſtneſs of reaſoning; ſince he ſeems to have built his theory on the fabulous ſtories of the ſettlement of Brutus the Trojan and Alboina the daughter of a Grecian king, in our iſland: and we know, from later examples, how unfit any one unacquainted with the Teutonic baſis of our language is for tracing its etymology and analogies.

ANOTHER ſubject, for which he was undoubtedly better qualified, gave riſe to his lateſt critical performance. This was the genuine pronunciation of the Greek and Latin languages. It is ſomewhat extraordinary that ſo ſoon after the revival of letters in this kingdom, we ſhould differ in our pronunciation of the learned languages from thoſe who were our maſters in them. This difference, we know, is at preſent very great. With regard to the Latin, we ſtand ſingle in our manner of pronouncing the vowels, in oppoſition to every other nation in Europe. Caius, by his long continuance abroad, and connexion with foreign literati, was led to prefer their method. As to the Greek, he wiſhed to have it pronounced after the manner of the modern Greeks, and not according

to

to that introduced by Sir John Cheke, which, however, is agreed to be in all probability nearer to the original practice. His arguments in support of these opinions are not very conclusive; and this piece of his, though short, is prolix and trifling. It was not printed till the year after his death; and was reprinted together with some others of his small works, by Dr. Jebb, in 1729.

I SHALL conclude this part of his character by observing that his Latin style is remarkably pure and copious, and formed upon the best models of antiquity.

OUR author's thorough acquaintance with the works of Galen will entitle him to all the medical knowledge of the age, which was circumscribed within the limits of that physician's voluminous writings. For him, Caius expressed the profoundest esteem and veneration; and from a person thus prepossessed in favour of a particular master, we are not to expect many new experiments or discoveries in his profession. The original works in medicine which he has left will, upon the whole, confirm this remark.

THE first, indeed, which he published can scarcely merit that appellation. It is entitled *De Medendi Methodo*, in two books, dedicated to Dr. Butts, physician to the king. It was drawn up during his abode in Italy, and printed at Basil in 1544. This is a general system of the practice of physic, formed upon the principles of his preceptor Baptista Montanus, and of Galen. He labours hard, however, in his own account of the work, to prove that it is not to be considered as a mere transcript; adducing a multitude of examples to shew that the most eminent authors have been imitators, without losing their title to originality. He claims the merit of arranging, selecting, and cloathing in more correct language the ideas of his preceptor; and ingeniously says, "Verba (ejus) expendimus, non numeravimus." He also asserts that some things in his work are entirely his own. "Nam ut plura Galeno quam a Montano accepta sunt, ita quædam ex nostra officina

"officina (ut de me modeſtius loquar) certe "promanarunt."

THE next of his medical performances is, however, indiſputably original; and the ſubject of it forms ſo curious an article in the annals of medicine, that we ſhall dwell upon it conſiderably at length. This is his account of the *Sweating Sickneſs*, or, as he named it, the *Ephemera Britannica*. Being a witneſs, during his reſidence at Shrewſbury in 1551, to the dreadful ravages made by this diſeaſe, he haſtily drew up an Engliſh treatiſe concerning it, deſigned for the uſe of the people at large. It was dedicated to William earl of Pembroke, and entitled *A Boke or Conſeill againſt the Diſeaſe commonly called the Sweat, or Sweating Sickneſs; made by John Caius, Doctor in Phyſic*, 1552, 12mo. This he ſome time afterwards reviſed, enlarged, and put into a more ſcientific form, and the Latin language; and publiſhed it in the year 1556, under the title *De Ephemera Britannica*. The dedication, to Anthony Perrenot, biſhop of Arras, is dated January 1555. It was correctly reprinted at London in 1721.

In this work we find the following account of the riſe and appearance of this extraordinary diſeaſe.

It began in the army of the earl of Richmond, afterwards king Henry VII. upon his landing at Milford-haven in 1485,* and ſpread to London, where it raged from the beginning of Auguſt to the end of October. It appeared in England four times afterwards at unequal intervals. In the ſummer of 1506. In 1517, from July to the middle of December. In 1528, during the whole ſummer. And, laſtly, in 1551, from April to the end of September. Its attack was extremely ſudden. It generally began

* Dr. Freind, in his *Hiſtory of Phyſick*, apparently tranſcribing his account of this diſorder from Caius, ſays that it appeared firſt in 1483, yet adds the circumſtance of its beginning in Henry's army at Milford. This he mentions as diſtinct from the viſitation in 1485. That this learned writer has here fallen into a miſtake, may be proved from our hiſtorians, who relate, that the earl of Richmond did indeed approach the coaſt of Cornwall with a fleet in 1483; but, on advice that the inſurrection of his friends had proved unſucceſsful, ſailed back without attempting to land.

with

with the affection of ſome particular part, occaſioning in ſome a ſenſe of a hot vapour running through the limb. To this ſucceeded extreme internal heat, unquenchable thirſt, and moſt profuſe ſweating. Anxiety, reſtleſſneſs, ſickneſs, violent pain of the head, delirium, and exceſſive drowſineſs attended its progreſs; and frequently in one, two, three, four, or more hours from the eruption of the ſweat, the patient was carried off. The violence of the attack was over in fifteen hours; yet the ſick perſon was not in a ſtate of ſecurity till the expiration of twenty-four hours; whence the diſeaſe is properly denominated by our author, an *Ephemera*. The perſons moſt liable to the contagion were thoſe in high health, of middle age, and of better rank and condition; children, poor and old people were leſs ſubject to its influence. The numbers carried off by it were incredible. In the town of Salop 960 died in a few days *(pauculis diebus)*; and our phyſician labours the deſcription of this calamity with all the ſtrong colouring of a Thucydides.

In his reaſonings concerning it, he firſt ac-

counts

counts for its being an Ephemera from the ſuppoſition that it attacked the more ſubtle ſpirits; whereas he conceives the plague and other fevers to attack the humours. He then proceeds to give his opinion concerning its origin and cauſe. He diſcuſſes the various ſources of contagion; conſidering ſeparately the effects of untimely ſeaſons, of noxious effluvia peculiar to certain places, and other contaminations of the air, and of planetary conjunctions. The immediate origin of the ſickneſs in his time he attributes to certain thick and ſtinking fogs riſing from the low grounds near Shrewſbury, which, being wafted by the wind, were perceived to carry the contagion with them. This general cauſe was, he ſays, augmented in particular ſituations by other ſources of corrupt air; ſuch as cloſe narrow ſtreets, dunghills, privies, uncleanſed drains, and the like. He ſtrongly inſiſts on the common notion of this diſtemper's being in a manner peculiar to the Engliſh; aſſerting that it ſpared foreigners, even the Scotch, in England, and ſeized the Engliſh in foreign countries. This he imputes to the greater luxury in diet by which our

our countrymen were, it ſeems, even then diſtinguiſhed from all other nations; and he confirms his conjecture by obſerving that the freeſt livers, and thoſe of the moſt athletic habits, were attacked with the greateſt violence.

THE method of prevention he propoſes is well ſuited to his ideas of the cauſes of the infection. It conſiſts in more abſtemious living, the uſe of acidulous fruits and ſauces, great attention to cleanlineſs, and free expoſure to the open air. He recommends the kindling of fires both round the houſe and within doors; looking upon fire as a great corrector of contagion, and adducing an obſervation to this purpoſe, that ſmiths and cooks were preſerved by their fires from the diſtemper. He directs aromatics and ſweet-ſcented herbs of all kinds to be burned in theſe fires, and alſo to be frequently applied to the noſe. He ſpeaks with ſome reſerve concerning evacuations, recommending gentle purgatives and bleeding only to the plethoric, and in them not later than the ſpring; ſince he thinks they ſhould meet the dan-

ger

ger in ſummer with a body undiſturbed and undebilitated by medicine.

The method of cure turns upon the ſole idea that the ſweat, from whence the diſeaſe is denominated, is critical, and therefore to be promoted in the greateſt profuſeneſs, till the danger is over. With this view, he directs the perſon ſeized to lie down immediately, in the cloaths he happens to have on, and have the body completely covered (all but the face) with bed-cloaths; in which ſituation he is to remain perfectly ſtill, not ſtirring a limb, if poſſible, nor putting a hand out of bed. He is to abſtain from food the whole twenty-four hours; and even from drink the firſt five hours. Then a little ale or beer, or wine and water is to be given in ſmall portions, and ſucked through a ſpout, the patient ſtill lying in the ſame poſture. At the expiration of about fourteen hours, the bed-cloaths are gradually to be removed, and the ſweating reſtrained; and after it is quite over, proper food is to be given to recruit the exhauſted ſtrength. This is the proceſs when the ſweat flows ſpontaneouſly. When this is not the caſe,

caſe, attempts muſt be made to excite it; and the means here directed are dry and warm friction, draughts of generous wine with *theriaca* or *mithridate* or aromatics, vinegar whey, China root, and other ſudorific medicines. By this method of practice, attentively purſued, and properly adapted to the circumſtances, we are told that the diſeaſe, though ſo fatal when neglected or miſmanaged, was got over with a tolerable certainty of ſucceſs; ſo that, according to Lord Bacon's obſervation, it might be looked upon "rather as a ſurpriſe of nature, than obſtinate "to remedies."

Valuable as this treatiſe of our author's is, not only as giving the fulleſt account of ſo ſingular a diſtemper, but as containing many judicious practical remarks, we muſt, however, acknowledge that it is far from a perfect piece of medical writing. It is not long, yet many digreſſions, foreign to the ſubject, are admitted; and trivial matters are dwelt upon more at length than thoſe of capital importance. Under the head of diet, the author takes occaſion to launch out into an enumeration of all the articles the tables of the luxurious at that time afforded. He employs ſeveral pages to deſcribe the methods of making beer and ale, and the proceſs of malting; and he concludes with a copious panegyric upon temperance, extracted from the antients. What we have moſt to regret, is the little light he affords us with reſpect to the firſt riſe of the diſeaſe; and I cannot but ſuſpect that he is guided merely by vulgar prejudice in ſuppoſing it ſo peculiar to this country. Its firſt appearance ſeems to have been neither amongſt Engliſhmen, nor in England; but among the foreign levies of the Earl of Richmond, who had either brought it with them, or, more probably, generated it in the crouded tranſport-veſſels on board of which they were embarked. This body of troops is deſcribed by a cotemporary hiſtorian (Philip de Comines) as the moſt wretched he had ever beheld; collected, we may ſuppoſe, from jails and hoſpitals, and buried in filth. A highly malignant and contagious diſeaſe might readily be produced in ſuch circumſtances; but why it ſhould appear under ſo new and ſingular a form,

form, why this ſhould be renewed ſo many times at irregular intervals, and ſhould at length entirely ceaſe, are queſtions perhaps impoſſible to be ſolved. That the climate of England was not eſſential to the exiſtence of that diſeaſe, is rendered manifeſt by its raging with great violence in Germany and the Low Countries in 1529 and 1530; and that the perſons of foreigners were not ſecure in England, appears from the death of Ammonius, a learned Italian, and a particular friend of Eraſmus, in 1520, (in which year the ſickneſs alſo prevailed in Calais;) and from the death of another of that nation, related by Caius himſelf. On the ſuppoſition of its being a fever of the putrid and malignant kind, we ſhall ſcarcely be able to account for its prevailing moſt among the rich and well-fed, contrary to what we now obſerve of that claſs of diſorders; and, indeed, the vaſt numbers related to be ſwept away by it, evidently prove its frequency among the loweſt ranks of people.*

* If 960 perſons were carried off by it at Shrewſbury in a few days, the greater part of whom were neither children nor old people, of what rank in life muſt the majority have been?

It

It may be further added concerning this piece of our author's, that he propoſes it to ſtudents as an example of that univerſal method which he has laid down in his book *De medendi methodo*; and it muſt be acknowledged a very good ſpecimen of the *order* to be obſerved in treating a medical ſubject, though not entirely ſo of the *manner*.

A book *De Thermis Britannicis* is mentioned by him as one of the lateſt of his performances. It does not appear to have been ever printed; but from his account, it was a treatiſe concerning the nature, uſes, effects and diſcovery of the warm baths in Britain; with a preface, in which he largely deſcanted on the natural advantages of our iſland, not only with reſpect to the production of the neceſſities, but the conveniences of life.

As a Naturaliſt, our phyſician appears in a very reſpectable light. He, like his cotemporary Dr. Turner, was a correſpondent and intimate friend of the celebrated Geſner; for whoſe uſe he drew up his *ſhort hiſtories of certain rare animals and plants*, which were tranſmitted

mitted to Gesner at different times, and inserted in his works. They were afterwards collected into one book, enlarged and corrected, and printed by W. Seres, London, 1570. At the request of this great naturalist, he likewise composed a *Treatise on British Dogs*, which, at first hastily and rudely drawn up, was sent to Gesner by way of an unfinished sketch. This writer, however, dying of the plague in 1565, it never appeared in his works, though announced to the public; but was afterwards published by Caius himself, greatly improved and enlarged, in 1570. Both this and the former treatise have been reprinted by Dr. Jebb. The method made use of in the account of British Dogs seemed so judicious to Mr. Pennant, that he has inserted it entire in his *British Zoology*; and from his respectable authority I add, that all our author's other descriptions of animals are proofs of his great knowledge in this branch of Natural History. Gesner fully acknowledges the assistance he received from Caius, and always mentions him with great respect. In return, Caius most pathetically laments the death of his friend, and launches out into a kind of funeral oration on this topic, in the middle of his book *De libris propriis.*

Our author seems very early to have had a propensity to Antiquarian studies; for he projected a history of his native place, Norwich, about the time of his leaving the university, but was prevented by other occupations from executing his design. This taste he resumed pretty late in life, on the following occasion. Queen Elizabeth paying a visit to Cambridge in 1564, the public orator, in a speech before her, extolled the antiquity of that university, to the prejudice of that of Oxford. This incited one Thomas Key, or Caius, a fellow of All Soul's College, Oxford, to vindicate the honour of the seminary to which he belonged, in a publication, wherein he asserted that it was founded by some Greek philosophers, companions of Brutus, and restored by Alfred about the year 870. This was too great a triumph to be borne by the Cantabrigians; and accordingly, our physician, at the instigation of archbishop Parker, steps forth, and in a learned dissertation, to which

which he affixed the ſignature of *Londinenſis*, aſſerted the antiquity of his own univerſity, and called in queſtion that of Oxford. With all the forms of antiquarian certainty and preciſion, he eſtabliſhes its foundation by one Cantaber, 394 years before Chriſt, and in the year of the world four thouſand, three hundred, and odd. Thus, after defeating the Oxford claim from the companions of Brutus, yet allowing them an origin as far back as from Alfred, he gains a priority of time to Cambridge of 1267 years! This piece was firſt printed in 1568, and afterwards reprinted in 1574, with the addition of a *Hiſtory of the Univerſity of Cambridge*, in two parts; one giving an account of its origin, antient ſtate, and the foundation of the ſeveral Colleges; the other containing a complete deſcription of it as it exiſted in his own time.

OTHER hiſtorical and antiquarian works which he compoſed, but which were never printed, are, a book *De Antiquis Britanniæ urbibus*; the *Annals of the College of Phyſicians*; and *Annals of Goneville and Caius College, Cambridge*. His treatiſe *De Libris ſuis*, inſcribed to his friend Thomas Hatcher,* from which our chief information concerning his writings is derived, was printed at London in 1570. At the concluſion of it he mentions a deſign, if his life was ſufficiently prolonged, to write the hiſtory of Norwich, and to correct all the works of Galen.

FROM the view here given of this author's numerous performances, he will appear amply entitled to the praiſes of learning, method, accuracy and diligence. But the oſtentatious diſplay of that learning in digreſſions foreign to the point in hand, and the application of that diligence and accuracy to trivial and unintereſting objects, will ſcarcely allow us to extol him for that ſolidity of judgment, and enlargement of thought, which conſtitute the man of genius.

THE following is the complete liſt of his works, drawn up by himſelf.

EX NOSTRA COMPOSITIONE

De medendi methodo, libros duos.
De Ephemera Britannica, duos.

* A PHYSICIAN, educated at Cambridge.

De

De Ephemera Britannica ad populum Britannicum, unum.

De antiquitate Cantabrig. Academiæ, duos.

De hiſtoria Cantabrig. Academiæ, duos.

De canibus Britannicis, unum.

De rariorum animalium atque ſtirpium hiſtoria, unum.

De ſymphonia vocum Britannicarum, unum.

De thermis Britannicis, unum.

De libris Galeni qui non extant, unum.

De antiquis Britanniæ urbibus, unum.

De libris propriis, unum.

De pronunciatione Græcæ & Latinæ linguæ cum ſcriptione nova, unum.

De annalibus Collegii Medicinæ Lond. unum.

De annalibus Collegii Gonevilli & Caii, unum.

Compendium Eraſmi libri de vera Theologia, unum.

COMMENTARIOS, SEU ANNOTATIONES

In Cornelii Celſi de Medicina libros octo.

In Scribonii Largi de compoſitione medicamentorum librum unum.

In Frammingami opera omnia.

In libros Galeni de administrationibus anatomicis novem.
In ejusdem libros de motu musculorum duos.
De sanitate tuenda sex.
De Ptyssana unum.
De parva Sphæra unum.
Ad Thrasybulum unum.
De ossibus ad tyrones unum.

EX NOSTRA VERSIONE, LIBRUM

De placitis Hippocratis & Platonis, primum.
De libris Galeni suis, unum.
De ordine librorum suorum, unum.
De Diæta in morbis acutis, unum.
Nicephori Callisti de confessione in orationibus, unum.
Chrysostomi de modo orandi Deum, unum.
Paraphrasis Erasmi in epistolam S. Judæ, unum.

EX CASTIGATIONE NOSTRA, LIBROS

De administrationibus anatomicis Galeni, novem.
De motu musculorum, duos.
De ossibus ad Tyrones, unum.
De compositione medicamentorum, decem & septem.
De

De simplicium medicamentorum facultatibus, undecim.
De placitis Hippocratis & Platonis, novem.
De medendi methodo, quatuordecim.
De libris suis, unum.
De ordine librorum suorum, unum.
De sanitate tuenda, sex.
De parva Sphæra, unum.
Ad Thrasybulum, unum.
De Ptyssana, unum.
De victus ratione in morbis acutis, unum.
De succedaneis, unum.
De septimestri partu, unum.
De humoribus, unum.
De brevi designatione dogmatum Hippocratis, unum.
De usu partium, decem & septem.
De locis affectis, omnes; additis argumentis singulorum.
De febrium differentia, unum.
De morborum differentia, unum.
De morborum causis, unum.
De differentiis symptomatum, unum.
De causis symptomatum, tres.
De morborum temporibus, unum.
De purgantium medicamentorum potestate, unum.

De his qui purgandi ſunt, quibus medicamentis, & quo tempore, unum.
De anatomia Hippocratis, unum.
De diſſectione muſculorum Galeni, unum.
De diſſectione nervorum Galeni, unum.
De medicina libros octo Cornelii Celſi.
De compoſitione medicamentorum librum unum Scribonii.

EX NOSTRA INVENTIONE, LIBRUM

Primum de decretis Hippocratis & Platonis Græcum.
De Comate Græcum, unum.
Hippocratis de medicamentis Græcum, unum.
Fragmentum libri ſeptimi de uſu partium Galeni Græcum.
Bonam partem libri de ſuccedaneis.
Et de Ptyſſana quod defuit.

WILLIAM CUNINGHAM.

THE following account of the life and writings of this perſon is given by biſhop

bishop Tanner. He was a physician in London, and resided in Coleman-street; and is much applauded by W. Bull for his knowledge in astronomy and physic. He also lived at Norwich in 1556—1559, as appears from a work of his, in which he gives a plate of the city of Norwich. He was a public lecturer in Surgeon's hall, London, in 1563. He wrote,

Speculum Cosmographiæ, sive de principiis Cosmographiæ, Geographiæ, Hydrographiæ, sive Navigationis. lib. V. London, 1559. fol. and 4to.

Two Letters between W. C. and John Hall Chirurgion, 1565, *touching the Cure of the Pox. M. S. Bodl.*

A New Almanac and Prognostication calculated for the longitude of London for the year 1566. Lond. 1566. 8vo.

An invective Epistle in Defence of Astrologers. This is frequently quoted in William Fulke's *Invective against Astrologers.*

GALE, in his *Institution of a Chirurgion* makes

makes mention of a work written by Cuningham, and intended for publication, on the venereal diſeaſe, called by him *Chamæleontiaſis*, from ſome ſuppoſed reſemblance between perſons afflicted with it and the chameleon. As this work never made its appearance, I ſhall quote that part of Gale's dialogue which relates to it.

" *John Yates.* And doth not he number " *Chamæleontiaſis* among tumours againſt na- " ture?

" *Thomas Gale.* Nothing leſs; for he ac- " counteth all thoſe tumours, ſwellings, knots, " ulcers, and ſuch like infeſting the body of " man, but as accidents, and no part of the " infirmity; neither laboureth he ſo much in " theſe, as in expelling the ſickneſs which " bringeth forth theſe accidents; for theſe are " to be removed without difficulty or great " travail.

" *John Yates.* I judge his new invented " way of curation to be extreme and dange- " rous to the patient; for both the fumes,

" unguents,

" unguents, and ſtrait order of diet with the " woods, are well known to be dangerous, " and yet many times doth not that which " they promiſe. But yet if his way be perfect, " it is more to be liked, and he worthy " praiſe.

" *John Feild.* His way is void of danger, " eaſy to the patient, exact alſo and perfect."

Dr. Cuningham wrote prefatory epiſtles to ſome works of Gale and Halle, which ſhew him to have been a man of conſiderable learning. For the ſhare he had in the works of the former, ſee his article.

WILLIAM BULLEYN

WAS born in the former part of Henry the eighth's reign, in the iſle of Ely; and was nearly related to a family of the ſame name at Blaxhall in Suffolk. He was educated chiefly at Cambridge, though Wood mentions

tions him as laying a foundation of the liberal arts at Oxford. Where he particularly purſued the ſtudy of phyſic, and took his degree of doctor, we are not informed. The principal ſource of information concerning him is his own works. From theſe we learn that he was a great traveller in Germany, Scotland, and eſpecially in his own country; the ſeveral products of which, particularly thoſe of the vegetable kingdom, he aſſiduouſly enquired into. In, or before queen Mary's reign, he appears to have reſided much about Norwich, making curious obſervations in the natural hiſtory of the place. He purſued the ſame objects in a longer reſidence at Blaxhall in Suffolk. He afterwards removed to the North, and was more permanently ſettled at Durham, where he practiſed in his profeſſion with much reputation. He had a property in the ſalt-pans at Shields near Tinmouth caſtle; and was a particular favourite of Sir Thomas Hilton, baron of Hilton, who commanded this fortreſs under Philip and Mary. Soon after the death of this perſon, Dr. Bulleyn repaired to London; where he had not long been arrived, before he he was greatly ſurprized by a charge preferred againſt him by Mr. William Hilton of Bidick for the murder of his brother, the Baron, who in reality died of a malignant fever. Upon this indictment he was actually arraigned before the duke of Norfolk, and the moſt unjuſtifiable means were uſed to procure his condemnation. He had, however, the good fortune to clear his own innocence, and detect the malice of his proſecutor. This happened in 1560. His implacable enemy afterwards hired ſome ruffians to aſſaſſinate him; and upon their failure, arreſted him upon an action for debt, and threw him into priſon, where he remained a long time. All theſe incidents, which are related by himſelf, appear not a little myſterious; but it is not worth while to ſupply the want of further information by conjecture. We know nothing more of his hiſtory, but that he became a member of the College of Phyſicians, and was in high repute for his learning and acquaintance with the antient phyſicians and naturaliſts. He appears to have been warmly attached to reformation principles in religion; and had a brother, who was a divine, and

alſo

alſo an occaſional practitioner in phyſic. Dr. Bulleyn died January 7, 1576, and was buried in St. Giles's church, Cripplegate, London.

THE writings of this phyſician deſerve notice rather on account of the information they contain relative to the ſtate of medicine in general in this country, than from any original obſervations or improvements ſuggeſted by their author; who appears to have been a man of more reading, than judgment or genius.

A BOOK of *Healthful Medicines*, which ſeems to have been his firſt attempt, periſhed by ſhipwreck.

HIS earlieſt printed work is entitled *The Government of Health*; of which the firſt edition in 8vo. is dated 1548. It is dedicated to his friend and patron baron Hilton, and has a wooden cut of the author prefixed. This is a very miſcellaneous piece, containing an account of all the articles of food, and their ſeveral properties, and the method of preventing

preventing and curing all diſeaſes, interſperſed with moral reflexions and admonitions, as well in verſe as in proſe. It was probably a popular book, as it went through ſeveral editions.*

A SMALL piece called *A Regimen againſt the Pleuriſy*, dated 1562, is put next in the liſt of his works; but we have no particular account of it.

THE title of his next and largeſt performance is *Bullein's Bulwarke of Defence againſt all Sickneſſe, Soarneſſe, and Woundes that doe dayly aſſault Mankinde.* It is ſaid to be "gathered and practiſed from the moſt worthy learned, both old and new;" and is dated March, 1562. My edition, which is not called a ſecond, is printed, London, 1579, fol. This work is dedicated to Henry Cary, lord Hunſdon; and the author mentions that it was chiefly compoſed while he was in priſon. It is divided into four parts. The firſt is *The Book of Simples:* the ſecond, *A Dia-*

* I HAVE not ſeen this piece, but take the account of it from the *Biographia Britann.*

logue

logue between Soreneſs and Chirurgery, cocerning Apoſthumations and Wounds: the third, *The Book of Compounds:* the fourth, *The Book of the Uſe of ſicke Men and Medicines.* All theſe parts will afford us ſome remarks or quotations.

The *Book of Simples* is an enumeration of the articles of the Materia Medica, chiefly compiled from the antients. Under the head of Water, the baths of Buckſtone are ſpoken of as having "done many and ſundry good "cures, both to the ſore and lame." This is the earlieſt mention I have found of theſe waters. Speaking of fruit, he gives additional proof to what we have before adduced, that gardening was not in ſo low a ſtate here at that period as ſome have repreſented. He takes notice of a delicious kind of pear growing in the city of Norwich, called the blackfryar's pear, thought to be the fineſt in England. He mentions cherries as very plentiful, particularly in Kent; and ſays he has ſeen very good grapes growing in ſeveral parts of England. A curious account is given of a kind of wild pea, growing ſpontaneouſly on on the ſea coaſt. "*Anno ſalutis* 1555, in a "place called Orford in Suffolk, between the "haven and the mayne ſea, whereas never "plough came, nor natural earth was, but "ſtones onely, there did peaſe grow, whoſe "rootes were more than three fadome long, "and the coddes did grow upon cluſters lyke "the chats or keys of aſhe trees, bigger than "fitches, and leſs than the field peaſon, very "ſweete to eat upon, and ſerved many poore "people dwelling there at hand, which els "ſhould have periſhed for hunger, the ſcarcity "of bread was ſo great." An odd miſtake which he relates concerning the exhibition of the herb Mercury deſerves to be noted by way of caution. The lord Wharton was accuſtomed to take this plant medicinally in his broth. In the abſence of his cook, an ignorant fellow who undertook the office ſent to the apothecaries ſhop for Mercury Sublimate, which he boiled in his lord's broth, and was very near killing him by the blunder. In ſpeaking of the Ebony wood, he mentions certain ſuperſtitious uſes to which beads made of it were put, being employed as charms for the cure of diſeaſes. Under this head he inveighs

veighs with great warmth againſt the ſin of witchcraft, affirming it to be "more hurtful "in this realm than either quartan, pox, or "peſtilence;" and lamenting that "damnable "witches ſhould be ſuffered to live unpuniſh-"ed, and ſo many bleſſed men burned." At the end of this book are ſome rude wooden cuts of chemical inſtruments and medicinal plants.

THE ſecond book opens with the praiſes of ſeveral Engliſh medical writers, all of whom have already found a place in theſe memoirs, except THOMAS PANNEL or PAYNEL, the tranſlator of the precepts of the *Schola Salernitana*. An alphabetical liſt of other eminent medical practitioners is given, in which ſeveral names of our countrymen occur, of whom I find no biographical or literary memoirs ſufficient for a ſeparate article. It may not be improper juſt to enumerate theſe. They are, Doctors Buns, Edwards, Hatcher, Frere, Langton, Lorkin, and Wendy, all of Cambridge; Doctors Gee, and Simon Ludford of Oxford; Doctors Bartley, Carr, Huyck (the queen's phyſician;) Maſters, John

John Porter of Norwich; Surgeons Edmunds of York, and Robert Balthrop; and Thomas Colse, Apothecary. The matter of this book is entirely chirurgical, and extracted from various authors. Towards the conclusion of it he gives a short account of his brother Richard Bulleyn's practice for the cure of the stone. It consists in the exhibition of aperients and diuretics, with the application of an emollient plaster to the reins, and a lubricating glyster every evening.

The *Book of Compounds* is a miscellaneous collection of *formulæ* both for external and internal medicines. There is nothing in this part so worthy of notice as the tribute of praise he offers to divers good ladies and gentlemen who benevolently employed themselves in curing their poor neighbours. It may not be foreign to the purpose of the present work to assist his laudable intention of comemorating these medical worthies by quoting the passage. "Many good men and women within this "realme have divers and sundry medicines for "the canker," (cancer, I suppose) "and do "help their neighbours that be in peril and

" danger, which be not only poore and nee-
" dy, having no money to ſpend in chirurge-
" rie, but ſome do dwell where no chirurgians
" be neere at hand. In ſuch caſes, as I have
" ſayd, many good gentlemen and ladyes
" have done no ſmall pleaſure to poore peo-
" ple: as that excellent knyght and worthy
" learned man, Syr Thomas Eliot, whoſe
" works be immortal; Syr Phillip Parris of
" Cambridgſhyre, whoſe cures deſerve prayſe;
" Sir William Gaſcoygne of Yorkſhyre, that
" helped many ſore eyen; and the Lady Tai-
" lor of Huntingdonſhyre, and the Lady
" Darrel of Kent had many precious medicines
" to comfort the ſight, and to heale wounds
" withal, and were well ſeene in herbs. The
" commonwealth had great want of them
" and theyr medicines; which if they had
" come into my hands, they ſhould not have
" bin written on the backſide of my booke.
" Among all other there was a knyght, a
" man of great worſhyp, a godly hurtleſſe
" gentleman, which is departed this lyfe; his
" name is Syr Anthony Heveningham (of
" Heningham, Suffolk.) This gentleman
" learned a water to kill a canker of his own
" mother,

" mother, &c." Towards the conclufion of this book the author gives a particular account of the cure of the venereal difeafe by Guaiacum; in the adminiftration of which, he fays, few men are to be compared to Thomas Glanfield, a fkillful furgeon in London.

The *Book of the Ufe of fick Men and Medicines*, contains rules for the adminiftration of purgatives, bleeding, &c. precepts concerning diet; obfervations on the effects of the paffions, on prognoftic figns, and variety of mifcellaneous matter. As refpectful as he has before fhewn himfelf to empirics of rank and quality, he takes occafion in this part to fpeak with acrimony of one John Prefton, or John of Stoneham, an old Suffolk quack, much reforted to at that time.

The laft and moft fingular of Dr. Bulleyn's publications is entitled, *A Dialogue both pleafaunte and pietifull; wherein is a goodlie Regiment againft the Fever Peftilence; with a Confolation and Comfort againft Death*. 8vo. 1564. It is dedicated to Edward Barret, of Belhoufe in Effex, Efq. at whofe feat part of it was

 written.

written. This is more heterogeneous than any of his other pieces. It is a dialogue of twelve interlocutors, in which one remarkable character, description, or story is started after another, with very little appearance of method or connexion. Several parts of it, however, are curious and entertaining, and show the author to have been possessed of a considerable share of fancy. Such is the description of a tablature representing our old English poets, Chaucer, Gower, Lidgate, Skelton, and Barclay. The scene of part of the dialogue is laid at an inn in Barnet, where a number of emblematical pictures supposed to be in the house, afford further scope for our author's invention. This, with several other circumstances in the book, show that he had the Canterbury Tales in his eye. The medical part is not above a seventh of the whole volume; it contains an account of the causes, symptoms, and treatment of the plague collected from various authors; and the particular occasion of writing it was the pestilential disorder which raged in England in 1563.* It may be observed that the general idea

* The preceding account of this piece is copied from the *Biograph. Britann.*

idea of this work, in which the dialogue arifes from a number of perfons retiring from the danger of the plague, is obvioufly imitated from the Decameron of Boccace; but, with much more propriety, he makes their difcourfe chiefly turn upon moral and religious fubjects.

RICHARD CALDWALL

WAS born in Staffordfhire, and educated in Brazen-Nofe College, Oxford, of which he became fellow. He went through his medical ftudies with great reputation; and after graduating, fettled in London, where he was admitted into the College of Phyficians, and created cenfor, in the fame day; and in lefs than fix weeks was made one of the elects. In the year 1570 he became prefident of that fociety. He is juftly entitled to the grateful remembrance of his brethren, by founding, together with the lord Lumley, a chirurgical and anatomical lecture in the College, for the ſupport of which a perpetual rent charge of forty pounds per annum was laid upon their eſtates. The royal permiſſion for this purpoſe was obtained from queen Elizabeth, in the twenty-fourth year of her reign. It was in the courſe of theſe lectures that, as will hereafter be more particularly obſerved, the true doctrine of the circulation was firſt made public by Dr. Harvey.

Dr. Caldwall died in 1585, and was buried in St. Benedict's church, near Paul's wharf, London.

He was the author of a tranſlation of the *Tables of Surgery*, written originally by Horatio More, a Florentine phyſician. It was printed after his death, at London, in 1585. From a prefatory epiſtle of E. Caldwall's, the editor, it appears that Dr. Caldwall left behind him a great many medical and chirurgical pieces in manuſcript.

JOHN

JOHN SECURIS

WAS born in Wiltſhire, and ſtudied with great reputation in New College, Oxford, in the reign of Edward VI. From thence he went to Paris, where he diligently purſued aſtronomical and medical ſtudies; the latter under the celebrated profeſſor Silvius. On his return, he ſettled at Saliſbury, and was much reſorted to for his ſkill in the practice of phyſic.

He publiſhed annual pieces, which he called *Prognoſticons*; which appear to have been a kind of almanacs, accompanied with aſtronomical predictions and medical precepts. Anthony Wood had ſeen two of them, for the years 1579 and 1580. To the latter was added *A Compendium, or brief Inſtructions how to keep a moderate Diet.*

He was likewiſe the author of *A Detection*

and

and Querimony of the daily Enormities and Abuſes committed in Phyſick, concerning the Three Parts thereof. Lond. 1566. This is a little treatiſe, wrote with learning and plauſibility, on the often repeated complaint of the intruſion of irregularly educated perſons into the practice of phyſic, and the preſumption of ſurgeons and apothecaries in taking upon them to act the phyſician. A peroration in verſe, addreſſed to the two univerſities, is ſubjoined. When the falſe and idle theories, in the knowledge of which the medical education of the ſchools at that time conſiſted, are conſidered, it will probably be thought that the public did not ſuffer ſo much from unlearned practitioners, as the regulars of the faculty repreſented. This work of Securis's, however, was thought to have ſo much merit, that it was reprinted in 1662, and publiſhed along with Record's *Judicial of Urines.* The author is not named in the title page, but is called "A Doctor of Phyſick in Queen Elizabeth's Days."

In this piece is a reference to one he had printed about the year 1554, with this odd title,

title, *A great Galley lately come into England out of Terra Nova, laden with Physicians, Surgeons, and Pothecaries.*

JOHN JONES,

THE little that we know of his hiſtory is, that he was either born in Wales, or was of Welſh extraction: that he ſtudied at both our univerſities, eſpecially Cambridge, where he took a medical degree; and that he became eminent for the practice in his profeſſion at Bath, and in Nottinghamſhire and Derbyſhire. He mentions curing a perſon at Louth in 1562; and the date of his laſt publication is 1579.

He was author of the following pieces.

The Dial of Agues. Lond. 1556.

The Benefit of the antient Bathes of Buckſtone, which

which cureth most grievous Sicknesses. Lond. 1572. This is dated from King's Mede, near Derby, and dedicated to George Talbot Earl of Shrewsbury, who had built a large lodging house at Buxton, and added other conveniences to the baths. The work contains very little concerning either the nature or history of these baths; but chiefly general directions, compiled from ancient authors, relative to the diet and regimen proper to be used with a course of bathing. He supposes a little sulphur, but not much of any mineral substance to be contained in the Buxton waters; and peculiarly characterizes them from their pleasant, delicate, and moderate temperature; from thence inferring their efficacy in depravation, diminution, and abolition of the action of the parts.

The bathes of Bath's ayde, wonderful and most excellent against very many Sicknesses. Lond. 1572. This is dated from Asple hall near Nottingham, and dedicated to Henry Earl of Pembroke. An adress is prefixed "to his friends, kinsfolk and allies of Bath, Bristol, Wells and other neighbouring places."

He

He begins his work with eſtabliſhing the ſame and antiquity of the baths of Bath, and gives a genealogy of king Bladud up to Adam. In his ſecond part, a good deal of learning is diſplayed on the cauſe of heat in thermal waters; which he, with Ariſtotle, ſuppoſes to be ſubterranean fire. The third chapter chiefly turns upon the Galenical diſtinction of things natural, nonnatural, and contrary to nature. The fourth is more proper to his ſubject, containing rules for the uſe of the Bath waters. He mentions drinking the water, as well as bathing; and recommends as much as the ſtomach will bear, the firſt thing in morning. The time directed for ſtaying in the bath is, for perſons of a hot temperament, weak and thin, from five to ſix in the morning, and the ſame in the evening; for thoſe of a contrary habit, two hours in the morning, and an hour and a half in the evening. Our author ſays he is the ſecond perſon after Dr. Turner who has taken notice of theſe waters. We have ſeen, however, that Bulleyn juſt mentions them.

A brief, excellent and profitable diſcourſe of the

the natural beginning of all growing and living things, heat, generation, &c. Lond. 1574.

A translation from Latin into English of Galen's four books of Elements. Lond. 1574. Quære—is not this the same with the preceding piece?

The art and science of preserving of body and soul in health, wisdom, and catholic religion. 1579. 4to.

GEORGE ETHERIDGE

WAS born in the year 1518, at Thame in Oxfordshire; and admitted a scholar of Corpus Christi College, Oxford, in 1534, of which he was made probationer fellow in 1543. In this university he pursued the study of physic, together with those liberal and ornamental parts of science for which that seat of learning has always been famed. He taught

taught Greek privately ſeveral years in the univerſity before the year 1553, when he was made Regius profeſſor of that language. This poſt he retained till ſome time after the acceſſion of queen Elizabeth, when, on account of his having been active againſt the proteſtants in Mary's reign, he was obliged to relinquiſh it. He likewiſe ſuffered much at this time from frequent impriſonments. He continued, however, ſteadfaſt to the Romiſh faith, in which he had been zealouſly educated; and for his ſupport purſued the practice of phyſic in and about Oxford, chiefly among thoſe of his own communion. He alſo took into his family, as boarders, the children of ſeveral popiſh gentlemen, whom he inſtructed in the rudiments of ſcience. In this ſtation he maintained a high character, not only for medical knowledge, but for ſkill in the mathematics, in Hebrew and the learned languages, in muſic and poetry. Leland the antiquary was his intimate friend, and has celebrated him in his verſes. He was living in 1588.

Besides various tranſlations and poetical works

works (of which one of the moſt remarkable is a verſion of the firſt book of the Æneid into Greek heroic verſe) he wrote

Hypomnemata quædam in aliquot libros Pauli Æginetæ, ſeu obſervationes medicamentorum quæ hac ætate in uſu ſunt. Lond. 1588. This is a ſmall piece, dedicated to Sir Walter Mildmay, with a prefatory epiſtle in Greek to the College of Phyſicians. Its purport is, to add by way of comment to the practical part of Paulus Ægineta an account of ſuch remedies as were principally uſed in his own time. Theſe, we find, almoſt entirely conſiſted of purgative, bitter, and emollient vegetable ſimples, with the compound electuaries and pills of antient invention; and his work is little more than a collection of preſcriptions of this ſort, accomodated to different diſeaſes. He takes notice of the *Sweating Sickneſs* that raged in Edward the ſixth's time, and remarks that few died of it at Oxford; which he attributes to the ſuperior purity of its air.

Sir George Etheridge, the dramatic writer, is ſaid to have been deſcended from the ſame family with this phyſician.

GEORGE

GEORGE BAKER

WAS a furgeon in London; furgeon in ordinary to queen Elizabeth, and mafter of the company in 1597. He was author of the following works.

A TRANSLATION into Englifh of the third book of *Galen De Compofitione Medica*. Lond. 1574, 8vo. and 1599, 4to.

On Oleum Magiftrale. A Method of curing Wounds in the Limbs. On the Vulgar Errors of Surgeons. Printed together, Lond. 1574. 8vo.

The New Jewel of Health; a work tranflated from *Gefner's Euonimus*. Lond. 1570 and 1599. 4to. This is a piece treating of the preparation of chemical remedies. The title of the edition in 1599 is *The Practife of the New and Old Phificke*. It is full of wooden cuts of chemical inftruments, and is dedicated to the countefs of Oxford.

A PREFACE to *Gerrard's Herbal.* Lond. 1597 and 1636.

An Antidotary of select Medicines. Lond. 1579. 4to.

On the Nature and Properties of Quicksilver, inserted in Clowes's Treatise on the Lues Venerea, 1584. This is entirely extracted from other authors; as, indeed, all his works seem to have been.

HE corrected an old translation of *Guido's Questions in Chirurgery,* and Barth. Tracy's translation of *Vigo's Chirurgical Works*; the former of which was reprinted in 1579, the latter in 1586.

JOHNSON, in the preface to his translation of Ambrose Parey's Works, says, that "G. "Baker, surgeon in London, translated the "apology and voyages of Parey, since which, "as he hears, he is dead beyond sea."

JOHN

JOHN BANISTER, OR BANESTER

WAS defcended from parents of good condition, but in what part of the kingdom they lived, we are not informed. He ftudied at Oxford; and after applying for fome time to the fundamental parts of fcience, he entered on the phyfic line. In 1573 he took a batchelor's degree, and obtained a licenfe from the univerfity to practife; and fettling about that time at Nottingham, he refided there many years in great reputation both as a phyfician and a furgeon. His fame appears to have been at the higheft about the middle of queen Elizabeth's reign. When or where he died is unknown; but it was probably at London, as there was a long memorial of him in St. Olave's church, Silver-ftreet. From an epiftle of Clowes's, prefixed to one of Banifter's works, it appears that they both were at the fame time in the fervice of the earl of Warwick. He was author of the following works.

A needful, new, and necessary Treatise of Chirurgery, briefly comprehending the general and particular Cure of Ulcers. Lond. 1575. 8vo. This is dedicated to Thomas Stanhope, Esq. high sheriff of Nottinghamshire. The substance of the work is extracted from various authors, antient and modern; particularly Galen, Calmetius, and Tagaltius. It is by no means devoid of learning and method; but contains no improvement of theory or practice which can be cited as the writer's own. Several recipes of topical medicines of his own invention are indeed subjoined, but it is well understood at present how little merit there is in multiplying compound formulæ, to the number of which every practitioner may add at pleasure.

The History of Man, sucked from the Sap of the most approved Anatomists: Nine Books. Lond. 1578. fol. Of this piece, Dr. Douglas, in his *Bibliographia Anatomica*, says, "Opus "hocce duabus figuris sceleti humani ac to- "tidem partium externarum a Vesalio de- "sumptis, sed misere depravatis, ornatur."

Compen-

Compendious Chirurgery; gathered and tranſlated eſpecially out of Wecker. Lond. 1585. 12mo. This is not a mere tranſlation; but at the end of each chapter annotations are added, in which the author's errors are frequently corrected, and his deficiencies ſupplied from other writers, or the tranſlator's own experience, with conſiderable learning and judgment. Indeed, Wecker was an author who greatly required ſuch an annotator, being a ſervile copyiſt of the antients, without reflexion or method. One of the moſt important corrections made by Baniſter, is his declaration againſt the uſe of cauſtic applications in punctures, and ſtitching in inciſed wounds, of the tendons, which Wecker had recommended.

Antidotary Chirurgical, containing Variety of all Sorts of Medicines, &c. Lond. 1589. 8vo. This is dedicated to the earl of Warwick. It is a large collection of chirurgical formulæ, gathered out of various authors, with the addition of ſeveral of his own, and of cotemporary Engliſh ſurgeons. Some of theſe laſt are of an elegant ſimplicity, and are in general leſs compound than thoſe of foreign practitioners. Thoſe of Balthrop are among the beſt.

Banister's chirurgical works were collected into ſix books after his death, and printed at London in 1633, in 4to.

WALTER BALEY

WAS born in 1529 at Portſham in Dorſetſhire, and educated at Wincheſter ſchool. He was admitted perpetual fellow of New College, Oxford, after two years probationſhip, in 1550; and entering upon the phyſic line, was licenſed to practiſe in 1558, while he was proctor of the univerſity. About the ſame time he was made a prebendary in the cathedral of Wells, which office he reſigned in 1579. In 1561 he was appointed Queen's profeſſor of phyſic in Oxford, and two years afterwards took his degree of Doctor. At length he became phyſician to queen Elizabeth,

beth, and had a large ſhare of medical practice. He died March 3, 1592, aged 63, and was buried in the chapel of New College.

He is the author of

A Diſcourſe of Three Kinds of Pepper in common Uſe, printed 1588. 8vo.

A brief Treatiſe of the Preſervation of the Eye-ſight; printed firſt in the reign of Elizabeth, and reprinted in 1616 and 1654, and likewiſe in 1622, along with *Baniſter's Breviary and the* 113 *Diſeaſes of the Eyes*. It is a compilation chiefly from the antients; and with a few good rules, contains many fanciful and idle notions concerning the *juvantia* and *lædentia* of the eyes, with extraordinary recommendations of the herb *Eye-bright*. To the edition of 1616 is added a ſecond *Treatiſe of the Eye-ſight*, collected from Fernelius and Riolanus.

Directions for Health, natural and artificial, with Medicines for all Diſeaſes of the Eyes, printed 1626. 4to.

A brief Discourse of certain Medicinal Waters in the County of Warwick near Newnam. 1587. 12mo.

In the library of Robert earl of Aylesbury was a M. S. of our author's, entitled *Explicatio Galeni de potu convalescentium & senum, & præcipué de nostræ Alæ & Biriæ paratione.*

THOMAS MOUFET, or MUFFETT

WAS born in London; and in that city received the rudiments of learning. After spending some time at Cambridge, he travelled through several countries in Europe, and contracted an acquaintance with many of the most eminent foreign physicians and chemists, whose opinions he imbibed. He took the degree of doctor abroad; and on his return practised in his native city with great reputation. He resided for some time at Ipswich. He was particularly patronized by Peregrine Bertie, lord Willoughby, whom he accompanied

panied in his journey to carry the king of Denmark the enſigns of the order of the Garter. He mentions having been in camp with the earl of Eſſex in Normandy; which muſt probably have been in 1591. The latter part of his life he paſſed much at Bulbridge, near Wilton, in Wilts, in the capacity of a retainer to the Pembroke family, from which he received an annual penſion, chiefly by the favour of that celebrated lady, Mary, counteſs of Pembroke. In this retirement he died about the end of queen Elizabeth's reign. He had an elder brother who reſided at Aldham hall in Eſſex.

Dr. Moufet was a writer of conſiderable note; and appears to have been one of the earlieſt introducers of chemical medicines in England. The title of his firſt publication is

De jure & præſtantia Chemicorum Medicamentorum, Dialogus Apologeticus. Francof. 1584. This is an acute well-written apology for the chemical ſect in medicine, which then began to prevail greatly in Germany and other countries, but met with violent oppoſition. The dialogue is a kind of diſputation between a Chemiſt a Chemiſt and a Galeniſt; the latter of whom, however, is very willing to be convinced. The Chemiſt enumerates many eminent men who favoured his ſect; among whom are Montanus, Fernelius, Villanovanus, Fracaſtorius, Cardan, Geſner, Platerus, and Severinus. He enters into an explanation of the Paracelſian doctrine of the double life in animals, one, which acts in themſelves, the other, which acts upon other bodies; which doctrine ſeems only to be an extenſion of the word life, to ſignify every thing that is capable of agency. He then defends the chemical practice of extracting by means of menſtrua or the action of fire the active parts of vegetable ſimples; and falls into a keen raillery of the Galenical compounds, and the loads of nauſeous drugs exhibited by that ſect of phyſicians. To theſe he propoſes the ſubſtitution of tinctures and eſſential oils. He next conſiders the mineral claſs of medicines, and defends their uſe againſt the objections of the Galeniſt, proving that both antients and moderns of their own ſchool employed ſuch of them as they were acquainted with. Here are ſome very odd names of chemical noſtrums

noſtrums of different authors introduced; as *Oſtruthium*, *Thielæum*, *Oxylæum*, *Orionium*, *Pactolus*, *Turtur*, *Aquila*, and *Draco*. He argues ſenſibly againſt the objections drawn from the corroſive and violent nature of ſome chemical medicines, particularly oil of Vitriol, Mercury, and Antimony. Theſe are the principal matters treated of in this ſhort work; which exhibits a good deal of learning, and ſkill in argumentation.

To this piece, in the *Theatrum Chemicum*, 1602, are ſubjoined

Epiſtolæ quinque Medicinales, ab eodem Auctore conſcriptæ. They are all dated from London in the years 1582, 83, and 84. The firſt of theſe contains a defence of Paracelſus, intermixed with ſome keen reflexions on Hippocrates, Galen, and their followers. The ſecond expoſes ſome of the fanciful reaſonings of Galen, and maintains the propriety of reaſoning from the evidence of our ſenſes, rather than from imaginary hypotheſes. The third contains ſome very ſenſible and liberal remarks againſt abſolute ſubmiſſion to the authority of great

great names, or leaders of a sect. Here also are introduced some further attacks on antient medical doctrines. The fourth gives the application of the chemical principles, salt, sulphur, and mercury, to the phænomena of the human body, and the theory of diseases; and is a most striking proof how blind a person may be to nonsense and absurdities of his own sect, while he is sharp-sighted enough in detecting them in others. The last epistle treats on the benefits of foreign travel to a physician, and contains some exhortations to the study of chemistry. Padua is the medical school particularly recommended by this writer.

ANOTHER work of our author's is entitled

Nosomantica Hippocratica, sive Hippocratis Prognostica cuncta, ex omnibus ipsius scriptis methodice digesta. Lib. IX. Francof. 1588. 8vo. I have not seen this piece, but its title seems sufficiently to bespeak its nature. It may serve as an additional proof of the profound learning of the author; and will likewise shew how far he was from the folly and extravagance of some of the chemical sect, particularly Paracelsus,

Paracelsus, who treated with contempt the writings of the venerable father of physic.

The latest medical work of Moufet's is his *Health's Improvement; or Rules comprizing and discovering the Nature, Method, and Manner of preparing all Sorts of Food used in this Nation.* This was published, corrected and enlarged, by Christopher Bennet, at London, 1655. 4to. It is a curious and entertaining work, as well on account of the numerous anecdotes and observations quoted from the antients, as the information contained in it respecting the diet used in this country at the time he wrote. As to the practical part of it, though there are many good rules and maxims derived from experience, yet the want of just principles by which to estimate the nature of different kinds of food (a defect common to almost all dietists) and credulity with respect to facts related by old writers, render his reasonings of little value. It is somewhat surprizing that *he* should admit the fanciful distinctions of Galen founded on the qualities of heat, cold, dryness, and moisture; the fallacy of which he seems so well apprized of

in

in his chemical pieces. He was not one of thoſe rigid dietiſts who entirely exclude the pleaſures of the table; on the contrary, a cook might learn ſomething from his book, as well as a phyſician. His concluding aphoriſm certainly is not quite in the ſtyle of Cornaro. "If our breakfaſt be of liquid and "ſupping meats, our dinner moiſt, and of "boiled meats, and our ſupper chiefly of "roaſted meats, a very good order is obſerved "therein, agreeable both to art, and the "natures of moſt men."

SEVERAL curious obſervations in natural hiſtory are interſperſed in his enumeration of the ſeveral articles of diet; and our learned phyſician diſtinguiſhed himſelf more particularly as a naturaliſt, by enlarging and finiſhing, with great labour and expence, a work entitled

Inſectorum ſive minimorum Animalium Theatrum; olim ab Edw. Wottono, Conrado Geſnero, Thomaque Pennio inchoatum. This he left behind him in M. S.; and it was publiſhed at London in 1634 by Sir Theod. Mayerne, into

into whofe hands it came by means of one Darnel, who had been Moufet's apothecary. Some imperfect copies of it, however, had been printed by Laur. Scholzius in 1598. It was tranflated into Englifh, and publifhed in 1658. Haller, in his notes on Boerhaave's *Meth. ftud. medic.* fpeaks thus of this work. ——"Pro fua ætate fatis copiofus, fpecies "multiplicavit, receptis varietatibus, icones "dedit fatis bonas, defcriptiones nimis philo- "logicas, neque copiofas fatis, fabularum ju- "gum non excuffit, minime tamen fua laude "fraudandus, & Entomologorum ante Swam- "merdamium princeps."

SIR Theod. Mayerne complains much in an epiftle prefixed to this work, of the great difficulty he found in getting a printer to undertake it; feveral in various countries having refufed his offer.

WILLIAM GILBERT, OR GILBERD

WAS born in the year 1540 at Colchefter, of which borough his father had been recorder. He

He is ſaid by Wood to have been educated in both our univerſities; but his epitaph mentions only Cambridge. After ſtudying here ſome time, he travelled abroad for further improvement in thoſe branches of ſcience to which he was particularly addicted; and probably took the degree of Doctor of Phyſic in ſome foreign univerſity. He returned to his own country with a high character for philoſophical and chemical knowledge; and was made a member of the College of Phyſicians in London. In this city he ſettled about the year 1573; and practiſed with ſo much reputation and ſucceſs, that he at length became firſt phyſician to queen Elizabeth, in which office he continued during the life of that princeſs. The vacancies from the duties of his profeſſion he employed in the purſuit of philoſophical experiments, particularly relative to the magnet; and in theſe he was aſſiſted by a penſion from queen Elizabeth; a circumſtance which deſerves mentioning to her honour; and the rather, as ſhe was accounted ſparing of pecuniary favours, eſpecially in the encouragement of literature. We are informed of no other circumſtances concerning the life

life of this learned man, who died, unmarried, November 20, 1603, aged 63, and was buried in his native place, where a handſome monument was erected to his memory by his brothers. He left all his books, globes, mathematical inſtruments, and cabinet of minerals, to the College of Phyſicians. His picture, which repreſents him as of a tall ſtature and chearful countenance, is in the gallery over the ſchools at Oxford.

THE capital work of Dr. Gilbert, entitled *De Magnete, Magneticiſque Corporibus, & de Magno Magnete Tellure, Phyſiologia nova*, was firſt publiſhed at London in 1600, and has been reprinted in Germany. This is not only the earlieſt complete ſyſtem of magnetiſm, but alſo one of firſt ſpecimens of a philoſophical ſyſtem built upon experiments, after the manner ſo much inſiſted on afterwards by the great lord Bacon. It is copious, methodical and accurate, as might be expected from an author who kept his M. S. under reviſion near double the time recommended by Horace. He begins with relating all that had been obſerved by the antients and moderns on the nature of the magnet; and among the latter, mentions ſeveral of our countrymen, to whom both the variation and declination of the needle were known. The diſcovery of this laſt property, particularly, he aſcribes to one Robert Norman. Then, after having diſcuſſed the various names of the loadſtone, and their etymology, he devotes the reſt of the book to an account of its various phenomena and properties. Theſe he divides into the following heads. 1. Its attraction. 2. Its direction to the poles of the earth, and the earth's verticity and fixedneſs to certain points of the world. 3. Its variation. 4. Its declination. All theſe he illuſtrates by a multitude of experiments, and various diagrams; and he attempts to account for the whole upon the hypotheſis of the earth's being one vaſt magnet. Various practical inferences of importance to navigation are deduced, particularly the great uſe of the declination in diſcovering the latitude at ſea.

This work has been applauded by ſeveral men of learning and eminence; as lord Bacon, Dr. Hakewill, Sir Kenelm Digby, and Dr.

Barrow.

Barrow. The firſt of theſe, ſpeaks of it in the following manner: "Gilbertus noſtras, cum "naturam Magnetis, laborioſiſſime, & mag-"na judicii firmitudine & conſtantia, nec "non experimentorum magno comitatu & "fere agmine perſcrutatus eſſet, confinxit "ſtatim philoſophiam conſentaneam rei apud "ipſum præpollenti."

Franc. Bacon. Opera.

It would appear, however, from a paſſage in his epitaph, that its reputation ſtood higher abroad than in his own country. It is this. "Librum de Magnete apud *exteros* cele-"brem in rem nauticam compoſuit." Joſeph Scaliger, however, upon whoſe opinion our author had animadverted in his book, exerciſed the well-known ſeverity of his pen againſt it, repreſenting the work as no-wiſe equal to the expectations it had excited.

Dr. Gilbert's attention to the nautical art further appeared by the invention of two inſtruments of very ingenious mechaniſm, for aſcertaining the latitude of any place without the aſſiſtance of the ſun, moon or ſtars.. This invention was publiſhed in 1602 by Thomas Blondeville, in a book entitled *Theoriques of the Planets, &c.*

ANOTHER work of our author's, entitled *De Mundo noſtro ſublunari Philoſophia nova*, was printed long after his death, at Amſterdam, in 1651, from two M.S. copies in the library of Sir William Boſwell. The ſcattered papers compoſing it, were collected with a view to publication by his brother, and were by him dedicated to prince Henry; however ſomething prevented his intention, and it did not appear till the learned Gruter gave it to the public at the time before-mentioned.

THE deſign of the work was no leſs than to eſtabliſh a new ſyſtem of natural philoſophy upon the ruins of that of Ariſtotle, which he attacks with great vigour and ſucceſs. Like many others, however, he was more ſucceſsful in pulling down ſyſtems than building them. Some juſt conceptions are mixed with much extravagant hypotheſis, as abſurd as what he attempted to explode. He, in common with the great Kepler, ſuppoſed the heavenly

heavenly bodies to be all a ſort of animated beings, poſſeſſing an intelligent principle. His beloved Magnetiſm alſo comes into frequent application. On the whole, this piece ſeems not to have excited the public attention in any great degree, nor added much to the author's reputation.

JOHN HALLE.

DR. Douglas, in his *Bibliogr. Anat.* calls this perſon *Chirurgus Londinenſis*, and he entitles himſelf one of the Company of Surgeons in London; it appears, however, from his works, that he was, for ſome time, at leaſt, ſettled at Maidſtone in Kent. Clowes calls him "Maſter John Hall, chirurgion of Maid-"ſtone, a moſt famous man." From his picture prefixed to his book, dated 1564, *ætat.* 35, he muſt have been born in 1529. This is all I can diſcover towards his hiſtory.

He publiſhed, in 1565, a 4to. volume, containing a tranſlation of the *Chirurgia Parva* of of *Lanfranc*; a *Compendium of Anatomy*; and an *Hiſtorical Expoſtulation againſt Abuſes in Phyſic and Surgery.* In an epiſtle dedicatory to the Company of Surgeons, the author acquaints us that the *Chirurgia Parva* was tranſlated about two hundred years before, out of French into Saxon Engliſh. This tranſlation, he ſays, he has not only put into more modern language, but has rendered more correct by collating ſeveral copies of the original. It is followed by *an Expoſitive Table*, explaining in alphabetical order the difficult words, and the names and natures of the diſeaſes and ſimples mentioned by Lanfranc. This is drawn up with a good deal of learning and judgment for the time.

HIS *Very frutefull and neceſſary briefe Worke of Anatomie*, is a ſhort piece, chiefly collected from other authors, divided into three treatiſes, and deſigned principally for the aſſiſtance of practitioners in ſurgery. Two rude cuts, exhibiting a fore and back view of the body, with references for the names of the external parts, are ſubjoined. He calls his work a more uſeful and profitable one of the kind than

than *any* hitherto publiſhed in the Engliſh tongue; yet ſays that the *firſt* anatomical treatiſe in the Engliſh language was that publiſhed by Thomas Vicary, in 1548: what others appeared in this ſhort interval I cannot find.

His *Hiſtorical Expoſtulation againſt the beaſtlye Abuſers, both of Chyrurgerie and Phyſicke in oure Tyme, &c.* conſiſts chiefly of accounts of certain medical and aſtrological impoſtors, who viſited Maidſtone and the adjacent parts while Halle reſided there. From the ſpecimens he gives of ſome of their bills, and the relation of their artifices to impoſe on the credulous vulgar, it appears that quackery has been the ſame thing from its earlieſt date to the preſent time, excepting that the character of conjuror is not now ſo often annexed to it. The author ſubjoins to this *Expoſtulation* ſome ſober advice to regular practitioners, much better than the poetry in which it is cloathed; and concludes the whole with prayers for the uſe of ſurgeons.

Tanner ſays he wrote, beſides the abovementioned works,

THE *Court of Virtue*, containing certain godly hymns with musical notes. Lond. 1565. 8vo.

TRANSLATIONS of Bened. Victorius *De Curat. Luis Venereæ*, and of Nicholas Massa *De Curat. ejusd. per Fumigationem.*

Epistles to W. Cunningham, M. D.

Directions concerning the Composition and Administration of Medicines used in Chirurgery. All these last in M. S.

JOHN DAVID RHESE

WAS born at Llanvaethley in the isle of Anglesea in 1534; and after about three years residence in Oxford, was elected fellow of Christ Church College in 1555. Without taking a degree in this university, he travelled abroad, and was made a doctor of physic at Sienna in Tuscany. He acquired so perfect a knowledge of the Italian language, that he was

was appointed public moderator of the ſchool of Piſtoia in Tuſcany, and wrote books in that tongue which were much eſteemed by the Italians themſelves. On his return, with a high reputation for medical and critical learning of all kinds, he, notwithſtanding, buried himſelf at Brecknock, where he paſſed the greater part of his life in literary purſuits and the practice of his profeſſion, and where he died about the year 1609. His conſtant adherence to the Roman catholic religion was probably a great cauſe of his continuing in this obſcure ſituation.

His works are,

Rules for the obtaining of the Latin Tongue, written in the Tuſcan language and printed at Venice.

De Italicæ Linguæ Pronunciatione. Latin. Printed at Padua.

Cambræ Britannicæ, Cymeræcæve Linguæ Inſtitutiones & Rudimenta, &c. ad intelligend. Bibliam ſacram nuper in Cambro-Britannicum ſermonem eleganter verſam. Lond. 1592. fol.

THERE

THERE was likewiſe in Jeſus College library a M.S. *Compendium of Ariſtotle's Metaphyſics* in the Welſh language, by our author; in which book he aſſerts that this tongue is as copious and proper for the expreſſion of philoſophical terms, as the Greek or any other language.

SEVERAL other valuable tracts, which are entirely loſt, were written by Dr. Rheſe, who was accounted one of the great luminaries of antient Britiſh literature.

WILLIAM BUTLER

WAS born at Ipſwich, about the year 1535; and educated at Clare Hall, Cambridge, of which he became fellow. Without taking a medical degree, he ſettled at Cambridge as a phyſician, and in time came to be the moſt popular and celebrated practitioner of phyſic in the kingdom. The means by which he arrived at this eminence, were ſomewhat different from thoſe employed by moſt of his predeceſſors

predeceſſors in fame, but have been uſed to advantage by ſeveral of his ſucceſſors. It does not appear that, like Linacre or Caius, he made himſelf conſpicuous for critical, polite, or philoſophical knowledge; but he ſeems to have been bold and ſingular in his practice, and to have poſſeſſed a natural ſagacity in judging of diſeaſes; and, what was perhaps more than all, his manners were extremely odd and capricious, which, with the vulgar, generally paſſes for a mark of extraordinary abilities. The following incident, which is ſaid to have been the occaſion of his being firſt taken notice of, will ſerve to give an idea of his character; if, indeed, it be not a kind of travelling ſtory, as from the nature of the preſcription may be ſuſpected. "A Clergyman in Cambridgeſhire, by exceſſive application in compoſing a learned ſermon, which he was to preach before the King at Newmarket, had brought himſelf into ſuch a way that he could not ſleep. His friends were adviſed to give him opium, which he took in ſo large a quantity, that it threw him into a profound lethargy. Dr. Butler was ſent for from Cambridge; who, upon ſeeing

ſeeing and hearing his caſe, flew into a paſſion, and told his wife, that ſhe was in danger of being hanged for killing her huſband, and very abruptly left the room. As he was going through the yard, in his return home, he ſaw ſeveral cows, and aſked her to whom they belonged: ſhe ſaid, to her huſband. Will you, ſays the Doctor, give me one of theſe cows, if I reſtore him to life? She replied, with all my heart. He preſently ordered a cow to be killed, and the patient to be put into the warm carcaſe, which in a ſhort time recovered him."* Probably, however, it was not by ſuch remedies as theſe that he acquired his reputation; but by chemical preparations, which he is ſaid to have been the firſt who uſed in England. Other inſtances of his oddities are recorded; as, that it was uſual for him to ſit among the boys at St. Mary's church in Cambridge; and that, being ſent for to king James at Newmarket, he ſuddenly turned back to go home, ſo that the meſſenger was forced to drive him before him. Fuller paints this humouriſt in the following

* M. S. of Mr. Aubrey, in the Aſhmolean Muſeum, quoted by Granger in his *Biographical Hiſtory*.

ſtriking

ſtriking colours. "Knowing himſelf to be "the Prince of Phyſicians, he would be ob-"ſerved accordingly. Compliments would "prevail nothing with him; intreaties but "little; ſurly threatnings would do much; "and a witty jeer do any thing. He was "better pleaſed with preſents than money; "loved what was pretty rather than what "was coſtly; and preferred rarities before "riches. Neatneſs he neglected into ſloven-"lineſs; and, accounting *cuffs* to be *manacles*, "he may be ſaid not to have made himſelf "ready for ſome ſeven years together. He "made his humourſomeneſs to become him; "wherein ſome of his profeſſion have rather "aped than imitated him, who had *moroſitatem* "*æquabilem*, and kept the tenor of the ſame "ſurlineſs to all perſons."

Dr. Butler ſeems to have reſided conſtantly at Cambridge, though he ſometimes came to London upon particular buſineſs. Dr. Goodall has printed a letter from lord-treaſurer Burleigh to the Preſident of the College of Phyſicians, dated February 1592, in which, at the requeſt of Butler, he deſires that he might

might be allowed the liberty of practising physic in London, whenever called there occasionally, or coming up on private business. This the College granted, provided that if he came to settle in London, he would submit to the usual examinations, and pay the customary fees. We find he was consulted, along with Sir Theodore Mayerne and others, in the sickness which proved fatal to prince Henry; and it is reported that at the first sight of him, Butler, from his cadaverous look, made an unfavourable prognostic. He did not, however, as Fuller seems to represent, immediately get out of the way; but attended with the other physicians till the death of the prince. An instance either of the credulity of the times, or of the singular practice of Butler, is quoted by Wood, in his account of Francis Tresham, Esq. who, as an author relates, "being sick in the Tower, and Dr. "W. Butler, the great physician of Cam-"bridge, coming to visit him, as his fashion "was, gave him a piece of very pure gold in "his mouth; and upon taking out of that "gold, Butler said he was poisoned." This mode of trial must probably have been founded ed on ſuperſtitious notions concerning the qualities of gold; yet it is poſſible that a *mercurial* poiſon might affect the colour of gold put into the mouth.

Sir Theod. Mayerne records the following inſtance of Butler's extraordinary practice. A perſon applying to him who was tormented with a violent defluxion on his teeth, Butler told him that "a hard knot muſt be ſplit by "a hard wedge;" and directed him to ſmoke tobacco without intermiſſion till he had conſumed an ounce of the herb. The man was accuſtomed to ſmoke: he therefore took twenty-five pipes at a ſitting. This firſt occaſioned extreme ſickneſs; and then a flux of ſaliva, which, with gradual abatement of the pain, ran off to the quantity of two quarts. The diſorder was entirely cured, and did not return for ſeventeen years.*

Dr. Butler was ſuſpected of an attachment to popery, but, as Fuller thinks, falſely, ſince he left none of his eſtate to an only brother, who went abroad and turned papiſt.

* Prax. Mayern. p. 66.

He

He died January 29th. 1617-8, in the eighty-third year of his age. He was buried in St. Mary's church, Cambridge; and the following pompous, but elegant epitaph was placed over him.

"Gulielmus Butlerus Clarensis Aulæ quondam socius, medicorum omnium quos præsens ætas vidit facile princeps, hoc sub marmore secundum Christi adventum expectat; & monumentum hoc privata pietas statuit, quod debuit publica. Abi viator, & ad tuos reversus, narra te vidisse locum in quo salus jacet."

He never was an author, nor left any writings behind him.

WILLIAM CLOWES.

Of this person, who was one of the most eminent surgeons of his time, I find no biographical memoirs but what may be extracted from his works.

His

His maſter in the art of ſurgery was George Keble, who probably practiſed in London, and for whom he expreſſes much eſteem and gratitude. Clowes was for ſome time a navy ſurgeon; for he mentions ſerving on board one of the queen's ſhips called the Aid, when the emperor's daughter married Philip king of Spain, which was in 1570. He returned home ſoon after this; for one of his cures, wrought upon a perſon of Town-Malling in Kent, is dated the ſame year. From the relation of another caſe, it appears that he reſided at London in 1573. Here he ſoon came into reputation, as may be inferred from his having been ſeveral years ſurgeon of St. Bartholomew's and Chriſt's hoſpitals, before he was ſent for by letters from the earl of Leiceſter, general of the Engliſh forces in the Low Countries, to come and take upon him the care of the wounded men. This was in 1586; and he went, by command of the queen, together with William Godorus, her ſerjeant-ſurgeon. Whether it was before or after this period that he was appointed ſurgeon to her majeſty, we are not informed. In an epiſtle of his prefixed to a book of

Banifter's, he mentions, as a particular caufe of friendfhip to the author, that they both ferved under the earl of Warwick. He alfo fpeaks in another place of having been a retainer to lord Abergavenny. The lateft date in his works is 1596; at which time he feems to have been in full practice. There is a difficulty refpecting the time to which he lived, that it is not eafy to folve. Dr. Alexander Read, in his lectures at Surgeons' Hall delivered about the year 1631, fpeaks of him as then dead. "Mafter Clowes, who, "while he lived, was a famous member "of this company." On the other hand, Woodall, in his *Epiftle of Salutations* to the Company of Surgeons, prefixed to the edition of his Works in 1638, begins his addrefs to William Clowes Efq. Sergeant Surgeon to his Majefty, and, at prefent, Mafter of the Company. As Read's teftimony concerning his death cannot be difputed, Woodall muft either have copied his dedication from a former edition, or the Clowes he addreffes to muft have been another perfon, perhaps fon of our author.

THE

The earlieſt publication of Clowes's is entitled *A briefe and neceſſary Treatiſe touching the Cure of the Diſeaſe now uſually called Lues Venerea.* This was firſt printed in 1585. An improved edition was publiſhed in 1596, and it was reprinted in 1637. He begins with lamenting the frequency of this diſeaſe in England; of which he gives this proof, that in the ſpace of five years he had cured about a thouſand venereal patients in St. Bartholomew's hoſpital. His principal method of cure is ſalivation by unction, together with profuſe ſweating, in the utmoſt ſeverity of the old diſcipline. He alſo mentions turbith mineral and mercurius diaphoreticus as efficacious medicines; and gives many miſcellaneous formulæ of purging potions, diet drinks, fumigations, ointments, plaſters, cauſtics, &c. He has a chapter on the nature of mercury, which he ſuppoſes hot and moiſt from its fluidity; and another on the practice of embalming. He cloſes with a ſtrenuous defence of writing medical books in the vernacular tongue, adducing the example of many authors, both foreigners and Engliſh, in ſupport of the practice. Among the latter, he enumerates ſeveral perſons whoſe names have already occurred in this work; and beſides theſe, doctors Langton and Bright, and ſurgeon Jemeny. In the preface to this treatiſe, he mentions a work on the venereal diſeaſe by a Dr. Theredehere, a French phyſician, which had been tranſlated into Engliſh by William Martin, ſurgeon in London.

The next and moſt important work written by Clowes, is entitled,

A proved Practiſe for all young Chirurgians, concerning Burnings with Gun-powder, and Woundes made with Gun-ſhot, Sword, Halbard, Pike, Launce, or ſuch other. To the firſt edition I have ſeen of this, a recommendatory epiſtle is prefixed, dated in 1588; but the edition itſelf was printed in 1591. It was reprinted in 1596, and 1637. This piece conſiſts, like the former, of caſes and remarks from his own practice, and obſervations collected from other authors. The firſt tract begins with caſes of burns from gun-powder. His chief remedies are a liniment of common ſalt and onion-juice, where the ſkin is left on, and

and emollient ointments to the excoriated parts. A very elegant cooling lotion uſed by a good gentlewoman is mentioned, which is a whey of verjuice and milk. This may deſerve to ſtand at the head of the *Pharmacopea Anilis*. In the treatment of gun-ſhot wounds, he adopts, what is commonly ſuppoſed a more modern improvement, the uſe of mild, mucilaginous cataplaſms; and in the relation of ſeveral dangerous and complicated caſes of this ſort, he ſhews himſelf a ſkilful practitioner. Some inſtances of punctured nerves and tendons are mentioned, in which he diſapproves of very ſharp and irritating applications; though indeed, under the notion of comforting and fortifying, he uſes warmer remedies than the preſent practice allows. A caſe of a fractured ſkull, in which he applied the trepan in two places with ſucceſs, is related; and another, of both legs much ſhattered with a gun-ſhot, which, notwithſtanding, he cured without amputation. In a ſimple fracture of the thigh he appears not to have been ſo judicious nor ſucceſsful. The extenſion made was violent; the bandaging very ſtrict; and though a very confined poſition was ſteadily preſerved, the diſeaſed limb was left ſhorter than the other. He next deſcribes the method of amputating, in which there is nothing very obſervable except the ſuppreſſion of the hæmorrhage; which he performs with buttons of an abſorbent and mildly aſtringent powder, applied to the veſſels, and ſuſtained by bolſters of lint and tow, and ſtrong compreſſion. This, he ſays, never failed him, and though he was acquainted with the method of drawing out and tying the arteries, uſed by ſome French ſurgeons, he never practiſed it. The powder was his own invention, and a ſecret; which, however, he had communicated to ſeveral of his brethren, and here makes public. After the caſes, follow many recipes of oils, cerates, ointments, &c. ſome his own, but moſt of them collected from other writers. There are beſides two wooden plates of ſurgeons' inſtruments.

To the edition of this work in 1591 are added, the tranſlation of *A Treatiſe on the Venereal Diſeaſe by John Almenar*, a Spaniſh phyſician; and ſome *Aphoriſms* relative to ſurgery,

ſurgery, in Engliſh and Latin. The firſt of theſe pieces, he ſays, was delivered to him by a friend for publication; the latter he happened to find in M. S. among ſome old books of ſurgery.

ON the whole, Clowes appears to have been a very ſkilful practitioner of ſurgery as it was in his time; and even an improver of his art. His quotations from Galen and Celſus, as well as from many later authors who wrote in Latin, ſhew him to have poſſeſſed a competent ſhare of learning. His ſtyle is clear, and not incorrect. He ſpeaks every where with great reſpect of his cotemporaries of the profeſſion, both native and foreign; and very candidly acknowledges any inſtructions he received from them. Nor is he leſs ſevere upon empirical pretenders; many of whom, he laments, were entruſted to practiſe on board her majeſty's ſhips, to the great detriment of the ſervice. He relates a ſtory in one of his prefaces, which may ſerve to ſhew the credulity of the times, and the petty knavery of an impoſtor in low life. An old woman, who had made a practice of pretending to cure all kinds of diſeaſes by a charm, for the reward of a penny and a loaf of bread, was committed for ſorcery and witchcraft by ſome of the wiſe juſtices of the country, and arraigned for theſe crimes at the aſſiſes. The judges, not quite ſo credulous, told the woman ſhe ſhould be diſcharged, if ſhe would faithfully declare in court what her charm was. She confeſſed that it conſiſted entirely in theſe verſes, pronounced after ſhe had received her pay.

My loaf in my lap,
My penny in my purſe:
Thou art never the better,
Nor I am never the worſe.

IT would have been happy for mankind if quackery and impoſture had always been as innocent as this.

PETER LOWE.

FROM this author's work, entitled *A Diſcourſe on the whole Art of Chirurgery*, the following circumſtances of his life are taken.

HE

He was born in Scotland. He acquaints his readers that he had practiſed twenty-two years in France and Flanders; had been two years ſurgeon major to the Spaniſh regiment at Paris; and had then followed the king of France (Henry IV.) his maſter, in his wars, ſix years. In the title page of his book he calls himſelf doctor in the faculty of ſurgery at Paris, and ordinary ſurgeon to the king of France and Navarre. His book is dated from his houſe in Glaſgow, December 20, 1612. How long he had been ſettled there does not appear; but he mentions, that fourteen years before, on his complaining of the ignorant perſons who intruded into the practice of ſurgery, the king (of Scotland) granted him a privilege under his privy ſeal of examining all practitioners in ſurgery in the weſtern parts of Scotland. He refers to a former work of his, entitled *The poor Man's Guide*; and ſpeaks of an intended publication concerning the diſeaſes of women.*

His

* Mr. Pennant (*Tour to the Hebrides*, p. 134.) copies the epitaph of Doctor Peter Lowe, in the cathedral church-

His *Discourse on Chirurgery* is written in form of a dialogue between himself and his son John. It is dedicated to James Hamilton, earl of Abercorn; and a prefatory epistle to Gilbert Primrose serjeant surgeon to the king, and James Harvey chief surgeon to the queen, is likewise prefixed to the work. The latter he elsewhere mentions to have written several learned works in surgery. This book is a general treatise of surgery, as well operative as judicial, designed for the use of beginners. It is copious, plain and methodical; full of

church-yard of Glasgow. It gives an amiable picture of his character.

Stay, passenger, and view this stone,
For under it lies such a one,
Who cured many while he lived;
So gratious he no man grieved:
Yea when his phisick's force oft' failed,
His pleasant purpose then prevailed;
For of his God he got the grace
To live in mirth, and die in peace:
Heaven has his soule, his corps this stone;
Sigh, passenger, and then be gone.

It is dated in 1612, the same year in which he published his *Discourse on Chirurgery*.

references

references to antient and modern authors, and, indeed, more founded on authority than obſervation. It contains no improvements upon the common practice of the times, conſequently nothing worth notice at preſent. What he ſays of amputation may, indeed, deſerve quoting, as ſhewing the ſtate of the practice in ſecuring the arteries, at that time, particularly in France, where he learned his art. In amputation on account of gangrene, he recommends the actual cautery as the ſafeſt method, on account of the tenderneſs of the parts, which renders ligature inſecure; in other caſes, however, he ſpeaks of ligature as ſufficiently effectual, and in applying it, he adviſes drawing out the veſſels with an inſtrument, and then paſſing a needle round them, including ſome of the fleſh. This was Parey's ſuppoſed improvement upon the ligature of the artery alone.

THIS work appears to have been in eſteem; for the fourth edition of it was printed at London in 1654. To the end of it is added a tranſlation of the Preſages of Hippocrates into Engliſh, by the ſame author, dedicated to the archbiſhop of Glaſgow in 1611.

AMES

Ames gives the following title of another work of his. *Easy, certain and perfect Method to cure and prevent the Spanish Sickness. By Peter Lowe, Dr. in the Faculty of Chirurgerie at Paris, Chirurgeon to Henry IV.* Lond. 1596. 4to.

FRANCIS ANTHONY.

THE history of empiricism is closely connected with that of medicine: or rather is a part of it; since the greatest variations in the practice of physic, as well useful as prejudicial, have originated from that source. No further apology, therefore, appears necessary for introducing among our biographical memoirs, an account of some of the most noted persons who rank under the class of empirics; and in doing this, I hope a general disapprobation of the character, will not prevent a candid acknowledgment of what individuals may have really done for the advantage of the healing art.

FRANCIS

Francis Anthony was born in London, April 16th, 1550. His father was an eminent goldſmith in the city, and had an employment of conſiderable value in the jewel-office, under queen Elizabeth. This ſon, after being inſtructed in the rudiments of learning at home, was removed to Cambridge about the year 1569. In this univerſity he applied diligently to his ſtudies; and after taking his degree in arts in 1574, he engaged with ardour in the purſuit of chemical knowledge. It does not appear that, according to the cuſtom of the time, he went abroad for improvement in theſe ſtudies; but it is probable that he continued at Cambridge till he was pretty far advanced in life. He then came to London, and began to publiſh the reſult of his enquiries, which firſt appeared in a treatiſe concerning a panacea extracted from gold, printed at Hamburgh in 1598. With this noſtrum and other remedies he undertook the cure of various diſeaſes; but not having applied to the College of Phyſicians for their licenſe, he was ſummoned before the preſident and cenſors, to anſwer for his illegal practice. Of this affair, the following account is given by by Dr. Goodall; which I ſhall inſert *verbatim*, not only as intereſting with regard to the ſubject of this article, but as a ſpecimen of the method in which the College proceeded at that time in ſuch caſes.

"In the 42d (of queen Elizabeth) Francis Anthony, Maſter of Arts in Cambridge twenty-ſix years, and afterwards Dr. of Phyſic in our own univerſities, appeared before the preſident and cenſors; confeſſing that he had practiſed phyſic in London for ſix months, and had cured twenty or more of divers diſeaſes to whom he had given vomiting and purging phyſic; to others a diaphoretic medicine prepared from gold and mercury: but withall acknowledged that he had no licence to practiſe. He was examined in the ſeveral parts of phyſic, and found very weak and ignorant; wherefore he was interdicted practice. About a month after, he was committed to the counter priſon and fined £5. *propter illicitam praxin*, in that he preſcribed phyſic againſt the ſtatutes and priviledges of the college; but within a fortnight or three weeks he was by a warrant from the lord chief juſtice

juſtice taken out of priſon and reſtored to his liberty. Wherefore it was ordered, that the preſident and one of the cenſors ſhould wait upon the chief juſtice with a petition from the college to requeſt his favour in defending and preſerving the college privileges; upon which Anthony ſubmits himſelf to the college's cenſure, and begs their favour. Wherefore it was ordered that he ſhould forthwith pay to the treaſurer of the college the £5. due for his fine, which he promiſed to do, and was likewiſe interdicted practice. Not long after, he was again accuſed of practiſing phyſic, which he confeſſed, wherefore he was puniſhed £5. for practiſing againſt the ſtatutes of the college and his own promiſe; but he refuſing to pay it, was committed to priſon and fined £20. About eight months after, order was given by the cenſors for proſecuting him at law, he having confeſſed three years practice within the city, and his preſcribing medicines lately to one that died, and to another in great danger. After this, Anthony's wife petitioned the college that they would deal mercifully with her huſband, and reſtore him to his liberty. This petition was rejected, it being

no

now out of the college's power to ſet him at liberty, the ſuit depending being commenced in the queen's name as well as the college's. Wherefore about two months after, Mrs. Anthony delivered a ſecond petition to the college, with ſo great importunity and tears, that partly upon that account, and partly upon the account of Anthony's poverty, &c. they granted the following warrant to the keeper of the priſon."

(THIS warrant ſpecifies that they are willing to diſcharge their part of Anthony's debt, ſo that it be no-wiſe prejudicial to her majeſty's part, which was £30.)

"Two years after Anthony's releaſe from priſon, Dr. Taylor with two phyſicians more of the college and ſome other perſons complained againſt him for preſcribing phyſic to ſeveral patients, amongſt which one died upon the uſe of his remedies; another loſt all his teeth; a third fell into ſuch violent vomitings and looſeneſs, that the day after he died and charged his death upon Anthony, who had ſaid that when all other remedies failed

failed him, he uſed this as his laſt and extreme one, which in the nature of it would either kill or cure. The preſident and cenſors gave order for his proſecution according to law. After which order, ſeveral freſh complaints were brought againſt him; as his preſcribing his *Aurum potabile* to a reverend divine, who upon his death-bed complained that this medicine had killed him, he falling upon the uſe of it into an incurable inflammation of the throat, &c."

Goodall's Hiſt. Coll. Phyſ. p. 349, & ſeq.

WITH reſpect to our empiric's favourite noſtrum, his potable gold, he publiſhed, in the year 1610, a defence of it, in Latin, by no means devoid of learning and art, although, in the preſent improved ſtate of chemiſtry and medicine, it would be thought deſtitute of ſolidity. The work is entitled *Medicinæ Chymicæ & veri Potabilis Auri Aſſertio.* It is methodically divided into ſeveral chapters, in which he attempts to eſtabliſh the poſſibility of making a potable gold, the great medicinal powers of the mineral kingdom, the ſuperior virtues of gold, and the claim a preparation of that metal may have to be entitled an univerſal medicine. Like many other empirics, he affects a wonderful fairneſs and openneſs in diſcloſing the nature of his medicine, while he conceals the moſt eſſential circumſtance of its preparation. By this artifice, the author of his life in the *Biographia Britannica* has been ſo much impoſed upon, that he makes this abſurd aſſertion. "Herein the author very fairly and accurately "relates the whole proceſs of his AURUM "POTABILE, *concealing only the method by which* "*it is diſſolved.*" This writer, however, at the end of the article inſerts Dr. Anthony's entire proceſs, as faithfully tranſcribed from a M. S. which he left behind him. In it the chemical reader will find the moſt extraordinary blunders and falſities ever offered to the public. A ſaturated ſolution of calx of tin in diſtilled vinegar is to be made, which, however, is to be *diſtilled*; and the liquor drawn over, (though, as every chemiſt knows, it would be a mere phlegm) is the menſtruum. Then gold filings and ſalt are to be repeatedly calcined and ground together, when, upon elixation with water, all the gold will be found

found converted into a white calx; a phenomenon altogether new in chemiſtry! Upon this calx the menſtruum is now to be poured; and after digeſtion during nine days, the ſolution is to be decanted, and evaporated to the conſiſtence of honey. From this extract, reduced to powder, a tincture is to be drawn, with rectified ſpirit, which, again inſpiſſated, gives an extract, an ounce of which, put into a quart of Canary wine, is the *Aurum potabile*. Though this proceſs was probably not the real one; yet we find that many of the moſt celebrated recipes for potable gold were equally incapable of affording a ſingle grain of that metal in ſolution.

Dr. Anthony's book was not unnoticed by the regulars of the faculty. An anſwer was publiſhed the next year by Dr. Matthew Gwinne, of the college, entitled *Aurum non Aurum, ſive Adverſaria in aſſertorem Chymiæ, ſed veræ Medicinæ deſertorem, Fran. Anthonium.* Other attacks were likewiſe made upon the potable gold; which induced the inventor to publiſh in 1616, an Engliſh Apology *in defence of his medicine*. This, beſides a repetition of the matter in the Latin treatiſe, has ſome additions; particularly ſeveral popular arguments in favour of the idea of an univerſal medicine, and a large collection of atteſted cures. Few empirical medicines have been more reſpectably ſupported by teſtimonials than this; and notwithſtanding the well-known fallacy of theſe proofs, it appears pretty evident, that Anthony's pretended preparations of gold were really powerful chemical remedies. They were probably mercurial or antimonial; for, in deſcribing their effects, he mentions their operating at times as ſudorific, emetic, diuretic and cathartic. Opiates were probably joined, as they were remarkably efficacious in allaying pain and procuring ſleep. They were exhibited under three forms, which he calls tincture of gold, potable gold, and quinteſſence of gold. The firſt, diluted in ſixteen times its quantity of wine, made the ſecond. The third was the dry reſiduum of the tincture diſtilled.

In an Appendix annexed to this tract, the author makes ſome juſt ſtrictures on a paſſage of Dr. Gwinne's book againſt him, in which the

the king is requested to suppress the medicine, lest the business of the physician, surgeon, and apothecary should be entirely ruined. This would seem not only to shew that the opposition proceeded from selfish and unworthy motives, but that the efficacy of the medicine was really extraordinary. It appears too, that Dr. Gwinne included all chemical medicines in his censure.

Two of the cases published by Anthony, which seemed to affect the reputation of Dr. Cotta of Northampton, brought on a very severe attack from that physician, who, however, delayed the publication till the year 1623. But notwithstanding this, and the former opposition he met with from the college and individuals of the faculty, Dr. Anthony found means to engage the patronage of several persons of rank, and the good opinion of the public at large; to which the excellence of his moral character, and his learning and easy address, did not a little contribute. It is certain, that later empirics, with more absurd pretensions, and much less merit to support them, have been alike victorious over good ſenſe and modeſty; ſo that we need not be ſurpriſed at the triumph Dr. Anthony obtained, in ſeeing his reputation, practice, and emoluments arrive at a great height. He is ſaid to have been liberal in his charity to the poor, and to have lived hoſpitably at his houſe in Bartholomew's cloſe, where he died, aged 74, on May 26, 1623. He left two ſons, both phyſicians; one of whom ſupported himſelf handſomely by the ſale of his father's noſtrum, the other ſettled and practiſed with reputation in the town of Bedford.

RICHARD BANISTER.

ALL the information I can find concerning this perſon is derived from his works. He ſays he was educated under his near kinſman John Baniſter, before mentioned. That, however, when he came to conſider the large field of ſurgery and medicine, he choſe to confine himſelf to certain particular branches; as as "the help of hearing by the inſtrument, "the cure of the hare-lip and the wry neck, "and diſeaſes of the eyes." In order to improve his ſkill in theſe operations, he frequented ſome eminent perſons of that time in theſe ſeveral departments; as "Henry Black-"borne, Robert Hall of Worceſter, Maſter "Velder of Fennie Stanton, Maſter Surflet of "Lynne, Maſter Barnabie of Peterborough." With theſe, he ſays, he ſaw much practice, but little theory; in order to ſupply which defect, he betook himſelf to the ſtudy of the beſt authors, as Rhazes, Meſue, Fernelius, Veſalius, &c. Thus accompliſhed, he fixed himſelf at Stamford in Lincolnſhire, making excurſions, however, to the large towns round about. The great reputation he acquired may be inferred from the numerous operations for the cataract which his work ſhews him to have performed, and from his being ſent for even to London, which city he at length viſited for many years in ſpring and autumn. He mentions having cured twenty-four blind perſons at Norwich, of which he obtained a certificate from the mayor and aldermen. At the time he writes this account, the year 1621 or 2, he he ſeems to have been grown old, for he declares, that knowing it is not long to the period of his days, he means for the future to reſt at home. We know not how much longer he ſurvived.

WITH reſpect to the works of this perſon, there ſeems to have been ſome miſtake among thoſe who have mentioned them. The title of that in my poſſeſſion runs thus. *A Treatiſe of* 113 *Diſeaſes of the Eyes and Eye-lids; the ſecond Time publiſhed, with ſome profitable Additions of certaine Principles and Experiments by Richard Baniſter, Oculiſt and Practitioner in Phyſick.* Of this, the treatiſe on the 113 diſeaſes is a tranſlation from the French of Jacques Guillemeau, made by one A. H. and at its firſt publication dedicated to the elder Baniſter. Being out of print, it was now republiſhed by Richard Baniſter, with a work of his own prefixed, entitled *Baniſter's Breviary.* Of this we ſhall give ſome account. It is dedicated to Francis earl of Rutland, and a copy of recommendatory Latin verſes by Dr. Prujean is prefixed. He begins with a ſet of aphoriſms on the nature of viſion, the ſtructure

of

of the eye, and its diseases, which are defective in method, and replete with the false philosophy of the times. He then mentions many errors in the common and empirical treatment of diseases of the eyes, and gives his opinion concerning the proper remedies to be used. In this part are many useful observations on the abuse of sharp applications. Then follow several remarks on cataracts, particularly those of the imperfect kind, as they were usually reckoned; such as the milky, bloody, soft, and adherent. These remarks are evidently the result of much experience, and shew him to have been a good operator, and a careful observer. He corrects the common notion that cataracts will always ripen, or become of a proper consistence for depression, by age; and asserts that in the soft kind, where the operation at first appears unsuccessful, a little time will frequently clear the eye, and produce the desired effect. He shews that what had been termed a black cataract, was really a gutta serena; and adds some useful remarks upon this disease. Some poetry is interspersed in his work, particularly some curious pieces to expose the pretended cure of bad eyes by well-

well-water; ſuch as that of Malverne, Wellingborough, Stratford-le-Bow, Shirburn and Tunbridge. He cenſures a practice which then prevailed, of drinking a large draught of ale the firſt thing in a morning for the benefit of the eyes; and concludes with a brief account of the qualities of the common remedies for the eyes, as hot, dry, cold, moiſt, &c. in the language of the old herbaliſts.

MATTHEW GWINNE

WAS born in London, where his father reſided, who was deſcended from an antient family in Wales. In 1574 he was elected a ſcholar of St. John's college in Oxford; of which he afterwards became perpetual fellow. In 1582 he was made regent maſter, agreeably to the cuſtom of the univerſity at that time, and was appointed to read lectures upon muſic. After taking his degrees in arts, he entered upon the phyſic line, and practiſed as a phyſician in and about Oxford. In 1588 he was choſen junior proctor; and in September

tember 1592, was the firſt replier in a diſputation held at Oxford for the entertainment of queen Elizabeth. The following year he was created doctor of phyſic; and in 1595, by leave of the college, he attended Sir Henry Unton, embaſſador from queen Elizabeth to the French court, in quality of his phyſician.

On the foundation of Greſham college, he was choſen its firſt phyſic profeſſor, being one of the two nominated by the univerſity of Oxford, and having a further recommendation from lord chancellor Egerton. This happened about the beginning of March 1596. At the commencement of the lectures in Michaelmas term 1598, he began with an oration in praiſe of the founder, and the inſtitution, which, with another delivered in Hilary term following on the ſame ſubjects, was afterwards printed. In June 1604, Dr. Gwinne was admitted a candidate of the College of Phyſicians; and in the beginning of the year 1605, was appointed phyſician to the Tower. In the month of Auguſt, the ſame year, king James with his queen and the whole

whole court visited Oxford, and were entertained three days with academical exercises of all kinds. Among the rest the two following medical questions were proposed for disputation.

An mores nutricum a puerulis cum lacte imbibantur? *Negatur.*

An frequens suffitus nicotianæ exoticæ sit sanis salutaris? *Negatur.*

The respondent was Sir William Paddie the king's physician; and the opponents Dr. Gwinne and others.

It is well known how inveterate an enemy king James was to tobacco; our physician was therefore politic enough to express his sentiments fully upon that subject after the trial of skill was over.

In the evening of the same day, a Latin comedy, called *Vertumnus, sive Annus recurrens,* written by Dr. Gwinne, was acted at Magdalen college. The following account of of this piece is given in *Rex Platonicus.* "Sed a cœna ad ſcenam properandum eſt, qua loco ſueto principibus a Johannenſibus "repræſentatur *Annus recurrens,* fabula ſocco "comico, ſed pede tragico, tragicis enim "ſenariis ad novitatem ſcripta, ſcena in for- "mam Zodiaci exactiſſime efficta, & ſole "omnia dodecatamorii ſigna ſplendido arti- "ficio pertranſeunte. Cujus decurſu quatuor "anni tempeſtates, quatuor ætatis humanæ "progreſſus, quatuor humorum corporis va- "rietates, & ſi quæ uſpiam ſint varietates aliæ, "aut fortunarum, aut ingeniorum, aut am- "orum, aut ludorum, omnes delectabili har- "monia in theatrum productæ, & micro- "coſmo repræſentatæ, adoleſcente primum "academico, aliarum deinde omnium condi- "tionum varietatem experiente. Sed quid "ego iſta, quum ipſa jam e prælo emerſerit "feſtiviſſima comœdia? Incœpta eſt ſole "arietem ingrediente, finita quum piſces ſolis "igne coquerentur. Digna quidem quæ toto "vertente anno duraret; ſed ideo Zodiacum "ſuum feſtinantius ſol viſus eſt tranſiiſſe, ut "principibus multo iſtius diei tædio laſſis "quieſcendi otium concederetur."

In

In December the ſame year, he was admitted a fellow of the College of Phyſicians; and in September 1607, he quitted his profeſſorſhip in Greſham college, probably upon marriage. After this, he continued to practiſe phyſic in London with great reputation both in the city and at court. In 1620 he was appointed one of the commiſſioners for garbling tobacco; for his majeſty, full of ſuſpicions of this weed, and attentive to the health of his ſubjects, cauſed directions to be drawn up for picking and ſorting this commodity, in which one of the faculty was, among perſons of other profeſſions, to be concerned. He died, according to Wood, in the year 1627. Profeſſor Ward, upon the authority of his name being in the *London Pharmacopœa*, printed in 1639, aſſerts this to be a miſtake. But a learned phyſician of my acquaintance has refuted this objection, by remarking, that the Pharmacopœa of 1618 was ſeveral times reprinted by the bookſellers without a reviſal, or changing the names of the college members. He left behind him one ſon.

THE

The following works of his, publiſhed in his life time, are ſtill extant.

Epicedium in obitum illuſtriſſimi herois, Henrici comitis Derbienſis. Oxon. 1593, 4to.

Nero, Tragædia nova. Lond. 1603. Wood ſays this is ſomewhere recommended by Juſtus Lipſius.

Orationes duæ, Londini habitæ in ædibus Greſhamiis, A. D. 1598. Lond. 1605. Theſe are reprinted, together with *Oratio in laudem Muſices,* never before publiſhed, in the Appendix of Ward's Lives of Greſham Profeſſors.

Vertumnus, ſive Annus recurrens. Lond. 1607.

Aurum non Aurum, &c. This work has been already mentioned in the account of Dr. Anthony, againſt whom it was written.

Verſes in Engliſh, French, and Italian.

A Book of Travels.

Letters

Letters concerning Chymical and Magical Secrets.

Dr. Gwinne, in the preface to his two Orations, mentions likewise that he had by him some discourses, entitled *Elucubrationes Philiatricæ*; but it does not appear that they were ever printed.

The learned professor Ward, from whose account this article is extracted, gives the following elegant summary of our author's literary character. " He was a man of quick " parts, a lively fancy, and poetic genius, " had read much, was well versed in all sorts " of polite literature, accurately skilled in the " modern languages, and much valued for his " knowledge and success in the practice of " physic. But his Latin stile was formed upon " a wrong tast, which led him from the na- " tural and beautiful simplicity of the antients, " into points of wit, affected jingle, and scraps " of sentences detached from old authors; a " custom which at that time began too much " to prevail both here and abroad. And he " seems to have contracted this humour gra- dually

"dually, as it grew more in vogue; for his "*Oratio in Laudem Musicæ* is not ſo deeply "tinged with it, as his *Orationes duæ* ſpoken "many years afterwards in Greſham college." Theſe are indeed perfect curioſities in their kind, and worth peruſing, as complete ſpecimens of the *interlarded ſtyle*.

DR. ALEXANDER READ, in the beginning of his chirurgical lectures delivered in Surgeon's hall, mentions a "Maſter Doctor Gwyn of "famous memory, who has delivered many "learned diſcourſes on ſundry points in the "art of chirurgery out of this ſeat." Whether this perſon was the ſame with the ſubject of the preſent article, I cannot determine; but the period of time will not be unſuitable to that ſuppoſition, ſince Read firſt lectured in 1631, and Gwyn was not his immediate predeceſſor.

PHILEMON HOLLAND

WAS deſcended from an antient Lancaſhire family of that name; and the ſon of Mr.

John Holland, a divine, who flying from the perſecution in queen Mary's time, afterwards returned to England, and was paſtor of Much-Dunmow in Eſſex. Philemon was born at Chelmsford in Eſſex, about the year 1551; and after receiving the rudiments of learning at the grammar ſchool of that place, was ſent to Trinity college, Cambridge, where he was for ſome time ſcholar to Dr. Whitgift, afterwards archbiſhop of Canterbury. After going through the uſual courſe of academical advancement, he left the univerſity, fellow of his college, and M. A.; and was likewiſe M. A. of Brazen-noſe college, Oxford.

He ſettled in the city of Coventry, where he was made head maſter of the free ſchool; and in this laborious ſtation he not only attended aſſiduouſly to the duties of his office, but ſerved the intereſts of learning, by undertaking thoſe numerous tranſlations which gave him the epithet of *tranſlator general of the age*. As if theſe occupations had been inſufficient for the employment of his time, he turned his ſtudies to phyſic, and practiſed

in

in that profeſſion with conſiderable reputation in his neighbourhood; and at length, pretty late in life, became a doctor of phyſic in the univerſity of Cambridge.

He brought up a family of ten children with credit; was a great benefactor to the poor; and was ſo peaceable and inoffenſive in his temper, that he never was engaged in a law-ſuit either as plaintiff or defendant, though he met with ſome unjuſt treatment. As a reward of his regularity and temperance, he reached his eighty-fourth year in full poſſeſſion of his intellects, and with his eye-ſight ſo good, notwithſtanding the great uſe he had made of it, that he never had occaſion to wear ſpectacles. He died of old age in his eighty-fifth year, on February 9, 1636.

He tranſlated into Engliſh, *Livy*, *Pliny's Natural Hiſtory*, *Plutarch's Morals*, *Suetonius*, *Ammianus Marcellinus*, *Xenophon's Cyropædia*, and *Camden's Britannia*; and into Latin, the geographical part of *Speed's Theatre of Great Britain*, and a French *Pharmacopæia of Brice*

Bauderon. * To the *Britannia* he made ſeveral uſeful additions. His tranſlations, though devoid of elegance, are accounted faithful and accurate; and certainly afford a memorable proof, how much a ſingle man may perform, if his whole time be employed to advantage. From the date of his *Cyropædia* it appears, that he continued to tranſlate till his eightieth year. An epigram is recorded, which he made upon writing a large folio with a ſingle pen.

With one ſole pen I writ this book,
Made of a grey gooſe quill;
A pen it was when it I took,
And a pen I leave it ſtill.

Dr. Fuller obſerves, that " he muſt have " leaned very lightly on the neb thereof, " though weightily enough in another ſenſe." Some other voluminous writers are ſaid to have had the ſame whim, as John Bunyan and Matthew Henry.

* Printed 1639. Lond. fol. with a dedication prefixed to the College of Phyſicians from Henry Holland the publiſher, ſon of Philemon.

A Quib-

A QUIBBLING epigram upon his tranflation of *Suetonius* has been often retailed in jeft books.

Philemon with tranflations fo does fill us,
He will not let *Suetonius* be *Tranquillus*.

THEODORE GOULSTON,

SON of William Goulfton, rector of Wymondeham in Leicefterfhire, was born in Northamptonfhire, and became probationer fellow of Merton college, Oxford, in 1596. After applying himfelf to the ftudy of phyfic in this univerfity, he practifed for a time with confiderable reputation at Wymondeham and its neighbourhood. At length, after taking his doctor's degree in 1610, he removed to London, and became a fellow of the College of Phyficians, and afterwards cenfor. He refided in the parifh of St. Martin's near Ludgate, and was in great efteem, as well for claffical learning and theology, as for the practice of his profession. He died in the year 1632; and by an article in his will testified such a regard to the interests of medicine, as entitles him to grateful commemoration. This was a bequest of £200, to purchase a rent charge for the maintenance of an annual pathological lecture within the College of Physicians. This was to be read sometime between Michaelmas and Easter, by one of the four youngest doctors of the college. A dead body was, if possible, to be procured, and two or more diseases treated of, upon the forenoons and afternoons of three successive days. If institutions of this nature, have, by the more improved and regular state of medical education, become less necessary, we are not the less obliged to those who founded them at a time when they were more wanted.*

Dr. Goulston published the following works.

* The public, however, has very lately been indebted to this institution, for some ingenious pathological essays, delivered as *Gulstonian Lectures*, by Dr. Musgrave.

Versio

Verſio Latina, & Paraphraſis in Ariſtotelis Rhetoricam. Lond. 1619, &c.

Ariſtotelis de Poetica Liber, Latiné converſus, & Analytica Methodo illuſtratus. Lond. 1623.

AFTER his death, his intimate friend Thomas Gataker, B. D. publiſhed his

Verſio, variæ Lectiones, & Annotationes Criticæ in Opuſcula varia Galeni. Lond. 1640.

EDWARD JORDEN

WAS born in the year 1569, at High Halden in Kent, and probably educated at Hart-hall, Oxford. After completing his ſtudies in his own country, he travelled abroad, viſiting ſeveral foreign univerſities, and taking his degree of doctor in that of Padua. We are told of an adventure which he met with in his travels, that had like to have proved fatal to him. Being in company with ſome zealous Jeſuits, he undertook the

 defence

defence of the proteſtant religion, with ſo much ardour and ſucceſs, that they reſolved effectually to ſilence him, by breaking into his chamber in the night and murdering him. He was, however, apprized of the deſign by one of his countrymen, who happened to be among his opponents, and prevented its execution by a timely eſcape. On his return, he practiſed for a time in London, where he became a member of the College of Phyſicians, and was in great reputation for learning and abilities. An inſtance of his good ſenſe, and of the eſtimation in which he was held, appears in the following circumſtance. One Ann Gunter appeared to have a diſorder attended with ſymptoms ſo ſtrange and ſingular, that they were imputed to witchcraft. King James hearing of the matter, ſent for her to London, and put her under the care of Dr. Jorden, who ſoon found reaſon to ſuſpect her of being an impoſtor. Being confirmed in his opinion by certain experiments, he acquainted the king with it; and by proper management, his majeſty brought the woman to confeſs that ſhe had counterfeited her extraordinary fits at the inſtigation of her father, with

with a deſign of fixing the odium of witchcraft upon a female neighbour who had quarrelled with him.

Dr. Jorden removed after ſome time from London to Bath, where he ſpent all the latter part of his life, univerſally reſpected as well in his private character as his medical capacity. His marriage, which from the circumſtances probably took place after his removal to Bath, was brought about in a ſingular manner. He happened, upon a journey, to be benighted upon Saliſbury plain; when, meeting with a ſhepherd, and enquiring after the neareſt place of entertainment, he was directed to the houſe of Mr. Jordan, a hoſpitable gentleman of good eſtate in that neighbourhood. The doctor conſidering the ſimilarity of their names as a good omen, rode to the place, where he was kindly received, and proved ſo agreeable to his hoſt, that he gave him his daughter with a conſiderable fortune.

Our phyſician had a natural propenſity to the ſtudies of chemiſtry and mineralogy; and as theſe were the foundation of the fame he acquired

acquired by his *Treatiſe on Bathes and Mineral Waters*, ſo they were the occaſion of much prejudice to his fortune, by engaging him in a project of manufacturing alum. Where his works were ſituated we are not told; but a grant he had obtained from king James of the profit of them, was revoked at the importunity of a courtier in that monopolizing age; and though he made application for redreſs, he could not obtain it, notwithſtanding the king appeared particularly ſenſible of the hardſhip of his caſe. That this diſappointment was of a nature not eaſily to be forgot, may be concluded from a paſſage in his book, where, his ſubject leading him to treat of alum ſprings, he thus gives vent to his feelings. "Now I "come to allum (Indignum vox ipſa jubet "renovare dolorem) the greateſt debtor I "have, and I the beſt benefactor to it, as ſhall "appear when I think fit to publiſh the arti-"fice thereof."

The doctor had ſeveral children, four of whom arrived to years of maturity, two ſons and two daughters. The ſtudious and ſedentary life which he led, aggravating the diſeaſes he he was conſtitutionally ſubject to, the gout and ſtone, he died in his ſixty-third year, on January 7, 1632, and was buried in the church of St. Peter and Paul in Bath.*

Dr. Jorden publiſhed,

A brief Diſcourſe of a Diſeaſe called the Suffocation of the Mother, &c. Lond. 1603. 4to.

A Diſcourſe of Natural Baths and Mineral Waters. Lond. 1631. 4to. This ſoon went through a ſecond edition, and was afterwards reprinted in 1669, in 8vo. by Dr. Guidott, and again in 1673. It is a work of conſiderable learning and ingenuity, written in a clear ſtyle and judicious method. Much of it is extracted from other authors. Of what is more peculiarly his own we ſhall give ſome account.

In order to ſolve the difficult problem of the origin of ſprings and fountains, he has the following ſingular hypotheſis. Comparing the ocean with its ſhores, to a cup brim-full

* The above memoirs are collected from Dr. Guidott.

of water, he ſuppoſes, that as in the latter the liquor will ſtand higher in the centre, than where it is in contact with the ſides, ſo in the former, the level of the ſea may be proportionally higher at a diſtance from land than on the ſhore. From this poſition, he imagines the riſe of ſea water through the pores of the earth, ſweetened in its paſſage, and burſting out in the higher grounds in form of ſprings, may be accounted for on the principle of the ſyphon, or the tendency of water to riſe to its former level. Inconſiſtent as this explanation may be with the now eſtabliſhed laws of natural philoſophy, it will not be thought deſtitute of ingenuity; and the ſame character will apply to his hypotheſis of the cauſe of the heat in thermal waters. After refuting by proper arguments the uſual method of explaining this problem, he purſues the following train of reaſoning. Generation, he aſſerts, is not confined to the animal and vegetable kingdoms, but is extended to the mineral; in which, as in the others, it proceeds from a ſeminary ſpirit, acting by a ſort of fermentation. He adduces ſeveral inſtances to prove that this generation of minerals is is conſtantly going on in the bowels of the earth, and that it is attended with heat; and from this heat and generative production, he ſuppoſes both the warmth and the impregnation of the thermal mineral waters to proceed, the ſprings of which may be imagined to ariſe from beds of minerals in their fermentative ſtate. He labours to prove that this cauſe would be gradual and durable in its action, and attempts to anſwer ſeveral objections to his hypotheſis that would occur.

THE practical part of his treatiſe relates principally to the uſe of the Bath waters. Theſe he aſſerts to be impregnated with bitumen and ſulphur rendered miſcible by nitre. Their internal uſe had not become common in his time; and he ſays he cannot commend it as much as it deſerves, on account of their adulteration in the baths wherein they are received. When they are taken inwardly, however, he recommends them to be drank hot as they are pumped. He denies that they have any purgative virtue, and obſerving that it was the cuſtom of the guides to give them with that intention mixed with ſalt, he imputes

imputes their effect to the salt alone. It appears from what he says, that they were at that time used internally in a dietetic way, in making beer, broths, &c. What he says of their external application is much the same with the present practice, except that he recommends bathing most in the hot months, as May, June, July and August. The time of continuing in the bath which he prescribes, is an hour or less in a hot bath, and two hours in a temperate one.*

JOHN WOODALL.

FROM the works of this excellent surgeon, the following circumstances of his life are collected.

HE was born about the year 1569. In 1589 he went over to France, as a military surgeon in the troops sent by queen Elizabeth to the

* See the account of Jones's *Bathes of Bathe's Ayde*.

assistance

aſſiſtance of Henry IV. under lord Willoughby. He ſeems not to have returned at the expiration of his ſervice; for we find him, after this period, travelling through France, Germany, and Poland, in which countries, he ſays, for want of better and more beneficial employment, he was forced for his maintenance to practiſe in the cure of the plague. He lived ſome time at Stade in Germany, among the Engliſh merchants reſiding there; and was employed by ſome embaſſadors ſent to that place by Elizabeth, as their interpreter in the German language. On his return to England, after the death of the queen, he ſettled in London, and made uſe of his former experience in a cloſe attendance on the ſick, during the great plague which raged in the firſt year of king James's reign. He became a member of the Surgeon's Company, and about the year 1612 was elected ſurgeon to St. Bartholomew's hoſpital, and likewiſe ſurgeon-general to the Eaſt India Company. This latter office was a poſt of great truſt and conſequence, ſince he had the charge of appointing ſurgeons and mates to all the Company's ſhips, and furniſhing their cheſts with medicines

cines and every other neceſſary article. It was on this occaſion that he wrote his *Surgeon's Mate*; but in what year the firſt edition of that work appeared, I have not been able to diſcover. It cannot be doubted, from many circumſtances, that he was for ſome conſiderable time a ſea-ſurgeon, and made one or more voyages to the Eaſt Indies in that capacity; but at what period of his life this happened, cannot from his works be aſcertained. As he mentions but eight years for the term of his travels by land, a period of three or four years will be left to complete the time between his firſt going to France, and his return to England after the death of queen Elizabeth: and this might probably have been ſpent in the naval ſervice. We are informed that he was likewiſe ſent into Poland, on ſome buſineſs of importance to the ſtate, in king James's reign.

In 1626, when the naval forces of the kingdom were augmented, and warlike preparations were carried on with vigour, the charge of fitting out the chirurgical part of his majeſty's ſervice was committed to the Corporation

Corporation of ſurgeons, and by them to Woodall. The king, Charles I. on this occaſion augmented the pay of the navy ſurgeons, and gave a bounty, proportioned to the rates of the ſhips, towards furniſhing the medicine cheſts. Woodall at this time wrote his ſhort treatiſe entitled *Viaticum*, being a kind of Appendix to his former work for the inſtruction of the younger ſurgeons. It was written in 1626, and printed firſt in 1628. From this period we learn ſcarcely any thing concerning him, except that he was for a time maſter of the Surgeon's Company, and that he reached his ſixty-ninth year in 1638, when he collected all his works into one volume, printed in 1639, which, beſides his *Surgeon's Mate* and *Viaticum*, contained a *Treatiſe on the Plague*, and another on *Gangrene and Sphacelus*. At this period he complains that his ſight was weakened, and his faculties much impaired, ſo that he was incapable of writing all that he had intended. How much longer he ſurvived I cannot diſcover.

Woodall dedicates his works to the king, the governor and committee of the Eaſt India

Company, and the master and governors of the Surgeon's Company. In his epistle to the latter, he asserts, that for forty years past, no English surgeon but himself had published any book of the true practice of surgery, for the benefit of young practitioners. In the preface he gives a kind of short history of medicine, which shews him to have been a man of reading; and he adds a sensible and modest defence of surgeons prescribing diet and medicines to their patients in certain cases, urging, that as they are liable to be called upon to serve their country, in situations where the whole medical treatment must be entrusted to them, it is unreasonable to deny them, in private practice, the exercise of such knowledge as they are obliged to possess.

THE first of his pieces, *The Surgeon's Mate*, is here inserted in the third edition. Its general plan is, first, an enumeration of all the instruments, utensils, and medicines of a surgeon's chest; next, a brief description of their uses and qualities; and then certain separate chapters upon some of the most important parts of military and naval practice. The

The design was undoubtedly meritorious, and is executed, upon the whole, in an useful manner; but since the matter is chiefly accommodated to mere novices in the art, I shall only take notice of some of the most remarkable passages.

Under the head of instruments he mentions one of his own invention, called *Spatula Mundani*,* contrived for the removal of hardened fæces, collected in the rectum; and he has several good observations on the frequency and danger of this accident. He also, after a whimsical riddling introduction, describes an instrument for conveying the smoke of tobacco, or other substances, up the intestines; the idea of which, as it would seem, was likewise his own. In treating on gun-shot wounds, he falls into the bad practice of the time, in recommending sharp stimulant applications to obviate the supposed tendency to gangrene; and, what is extraordinary, he does not once take notice of *Clowes*'s express treatise on this subject. Indeed, he is by no means so liberal

* Quasi, *mundans anum*, or *mundator ani*.

of compliment to his countrymen and cotemporaries, as that author, very ſeldom even mentioning their names. In opening abſceſſes, he greatly prefers cauſtics to the knife; and diſapproves the exorbitant uſe of hard tents and corroſive applications in the cure of ulcers. He does not allow the uſe of circular rollers in fractures, the renewing of which would diſturb the limb; but in their ſtead directs ſplints and tape. He ſpeaks much againſt tight bandage, ſtrongly inculcates the idea that the cure of fractures is entirely the work of nature, and indeed treats this ſubject ſo ſenſibly, that we may readily believe his aſſertion, that what he ſays concerning it is derived from his own experience, not from the authority of others. In amputation he recommends tying the large veſſels, eſpecially thoſe of the thigh, if it can be done; but he ſeems to think that the ſurgeon will often be foiled in his attempts. In this caſe, as well as for the ſmaller veſſels, he directs buttons of aſtringent and cauſtic powders to be applied.

THE moſt valuable piece in this work ſeems to be his tract on the Scurvy, which, whether for

for accuracy in describing the disease, or judiciousness in the method of cure, has perhaps scarcely been since excelled. He defines the scurvy to be a disease of the spleen; and asserts its principal cause to be the long use of salt provision, together with the want of cleanliness, and proper change of apparel. He describes its symptoms concisely, but with much precision; and then proceeds to the practical part, in which he is very full and particular. The remedy to which he gives the first place is the juice of lemons, the extraordinary efficacy of which he several times insists upon. In want of this, he recommends various other acid vegetable juices and fruits; and where none of these can be had, oil of vitriol. A variety of judicious remarks and directions concerning medicines, diet, and external applications, occur in this treatise; of which I shall only say further, that they appear evidently to be the result of experience and careful observation, and are in great part confirmed by modern practice.*

He

* The very ingenious Dr. Macbride, in his *Experimental Essays*, has particularly commended this treatise of

He has a chapter on the virtues of Paracelſus's *Laudanum Opiatum*, which he peculiarly recommends in the dyſentery, and prefers to every other preparation of the kind. The work is concluded with ſome chapters on ſalt, ſulphur, and mercury, and their virtues, in proſe and verſe, and an explanation of chemical characters and terms. Though there is nothing in theſe but what he has extracted from other authors, it ſhews that he had made chemiſtry an object of his attention, probably during his reſidence abroad; as, indeed, he in part aſſerts.

His next work, entitled *Viaticum, being the path-way to the ſurgeon's cheſt*, is written with the ſame general deſign of inſtructing young practitioners, but chiefly with a reference to the treatment of gun-ſhot wounds. Under this head there is nothing, however, materially different from what is given in his *Surgeon's Mate*. There is added a deſcription of the

of Woodall's, and quoted a conſiderable part of it. He likewiſe takes notice of his merits in ſome other reſpects, and expreſſes his ſurprize that ſo few modern writers have mentioned him.

trefine,

trefine, an inftrument invented by our author, and which has now almoft entirely taken place of the trepan. He contrived the variation from this laft inftrument, not only in the manner of working, but in the conical fhape of the faw, which prevents its fuddenly bearing upon the dura mater when the bone is cut through.

His *Treatife on the Plague* is fcarcely worthy of the great experience he boafts to have had in this difeafe. It confifts chiefly of numerous antidotes and remedies copied out of other writers, and contains little of his own, except the recommendation of a mineral diaphoretic noftrum of his, called *Aurum Vitæ*, the preparation of which he keeps fecret. Atteftations in its favour, from the parifh officers of *St. Margaret's*, *Weftminfter*, and the mayor and juftices of *Northampton*, dated in 1638, are annexed.

His laft piece, *A Treatife on Gangrene and Sphacelus*, deferves more particular confideration, on account of an important innovation in practice which it is defigned to inculcate.

This is, amputation in the mortified, inſtead of the ſound part; a practice not new indeed, but at that time univerſally diſuſed. His ſucceſs in a caſe which would admit of no other kind of operation, firſt led him to the idea of it; and he purſued it to ſuch a length, that he affirms he had taken off more than a hundred limbs in the mortified part, and in not one inſtance did the patient die, or the mortification ſpread farther. As the intention in this method could only be to relieve nature from the burthen of a putrid maſs, and leave the immediate ſeparation of the ſound and mortified parts to her own efforts, it may be conſidered as an important advance to that which is at preſent eſteemed the moſt judicious practice; namely, deferring amputation altogether in mortifications, till the gangrenous diſpoſition in the habit is corrected, and a line of ſeparation is already formed between the living and dead fibres. Several uſeful general remarks on amputation occur in this tract. Among the reſt, there is the firſt hint in favour of amputating as low as the ancle in diſeaſes of the foot; for upon obſerving that perſons who had undergone the

the puniſhment of having their feet cut off in the Eaſt Indies, were able to walk very well after their ſtumps were healed, by putting them into caſes of bamboo, he expreſſes a wiſh that the practice might be imitated by ſurgeons, though he acknowledges he himſelf ſhould not venture upon ſuch an innovation.

It is worth mentioning, that he aſſerts that for twenty-four years, in which he has been ſurgeon to St. Bartholomew's hoſpital, not one perſon had died of a hæmorrhage from amputation; that four-fifths of theſe patients went alive and well out of the hoſpital; and that for the fifty years in which he has known the art of ſurgery, he never ſaw in England or elſewhere, the cruel antient practice of cauterizing the ſenſible and living parts at the end of a ſtump.

THEODORE TURQUET DE MAYERNE.

ALTHOUGH this eminent phyſician was born and educated abroad, yet the diſtinguiſhed place he for many years occupied among

among the faculty in this country, and the important changes which he principally contributed to introduce in our medical practice, will, I doubt not, sufficiently evince the propriety of including him among the subjects of these biographical memoirs.

His father, Lewis de Mayerne, was a French protestant, and a celebrated writer of history. He fled, on account of his religion, from Lyons to Geneva, in the year 1572; and in that city his son Theodore was born on September 18, 1573. After being instructed in the rudiments of literature at his native place, he was sent to the university of Heidleberg, where he remained some years; but upon attaching himself to the profession of physic, he removed to Montpellier, and there pursuing his medical studies, he took the degrees of batchelor and doctor of physic in 1596 and 1597. Having thus completed his education, he went to Paris, where he gave lectures in anatomy to the young surgeons, and in pharmacy to the apothecaries. The latter of these subjects led him to treat on chemistry, to the practice of which he had paid peculiar attention; and as in his medical

practice

practice he made considerable use of chemical remedies, he was soon looked upon as one of the most strenuous supporters of this innovation, as it was then termed. While this brought him into favour with Riverius, first physician to king Henry IV. who by his recommendation procured him to be appointed one of his majesty's physicians in ordinary; it likewise drew on him the enmity of the faculty at Paris, who manifested their attachment to Galen, by an indiscriminate abuse of all who attempted to introduce modes of practice not mentioned in his works. Quercetanus was joined with Mayerne as the object of their attack; and in 1603, one of the body wrote a book against these heterodox brethren, entitled *Apologia pro Medicina Hippocratis & Galeni, contra Mayernium & Quercetanum.* To this Mayerne published an apologetical answer; and the Galenists not only replied, but proceeded to thunder an academical interdict against the two delinquents. The favour of the king, however, rendered this a *brutum fulmen* with respect to Mayerne; for his majesty having, in 1600, appointed our physician to attend the duke de Rohan in his embassies

embaſſies to the courts of Germany and Italy, he diſcharged his office with ſo much reputation, that he roſe high in the king's eſteem, and was promiſed great advantages, provided he would embrace the Roman catholic religion. This, however, notwithſtanding the perſuaſions of the Cardinal du Perron and other eccleſiaſtics, he refuſed to do: the king, nevertheleſs, ſtill would have appointed him his firſt phyſician, had not the Jeſuits influenced queen Mary de Medicis to interpoſe and prevent it—a ſtrong inſtance of their ſuſpicious and meddling diſpoſition. Mayerne continued in the office of phyſician in ordinary to the king, till the year 1606; when he ſold his place to a French phyſician; and in 1607, an Engliſhman of quality who had been his patient, carried him over to England.* Here he

* Some incertainty attends the time of Mayerne's ſettling in England. Wood, in his *Faſti*, places the incorporation of Mayerne at Oxford, in the year 1606, and ſays he was then phyſician to the queen. On the other hand, Mayerne, in his dedicatory epiſtle of Mouffet's *Theatrum Inſectorum* to Sir William Paddy, ſays, that after the aſſaſſination of his maſter Henry

he was honoured with a private conference with king James, who appointed him firſt phyſician to himſelf and his queen; and from this period to his death, he appears to have been conſidered as the firſt perſon in the profeſſion in this kingdom. He was received into both Univerſities, and into the College of Phyſicians, and treated with the greateſt reſpect by theſe learned bodies. In the courſe of his practice, he had under his care, not only the whole royal family, but a great number of the principal perſons, of both ſexes, about the court; and ever maintained an unblemiſhed character for care, diligence, and fidelity in the diſcharge of his profeſſion.

One of the moſt important, and at the ſame time, moſt unfortunate occurrences during the courſe of his employment, was the fatal

Henry IV. he was called into England by letters from king James's own hand, who alſo ſent a perſon expreſsly to conduct him over. Henry was not aſſaſſinated till May 14, 1610. From theſe different accounts it appears probable, that he had viſited England and formed connections at court, ſome time before he came to reſide here.

ſickneſs

ſickneſs of Henry prince of Wales, the eldeſt ſon of king James, and the darling hope of his ſubjects. This prince was taken ill on October 15, 1612; but it was not till the 25th, that his diſorder was thought of importance enough to require the aſſiſtance of Dr. Mayerne, in addition to that of Dr. Hammond his phyſician in ordinary. The diſeaſe was a putrid fever; and the moſt accurate account of its progreſs, together with every circumſtance of the prince's conſtitution and manner of life which might prediſpoſe to it, is given in the collection of caſes left by Mayerne; who, from the time of his being called in, appears to have had the chief management of the caſe. The patient died on November 6, and from the whole courſe of the ſymptoms, as well as the appearances on diſſection, there cannot be the leaſt doubt that his death was the conſequence of a natural diſeaſe, and not induced by any iniquitous means, as ſome of the enemies of that unhappy family have affected to believe. We find, however, that certain malicious reflections, which were at that time made, againſt either the fidelity or ſkill of our phyſician

ſician in this affair, influenced him, beſides drawing up both in French and Latin a minute account of the whole diſeaſe and its treatment, to procure a certificate from the king, expreſſing the moſt perfect ſatisfaction with his conduct; and two others from the lords of the council, and the officers and gentlemen of the prince, to the ſame purpoſe. His diſagreement in opinion with the other phyſicians, with reſpect to bleeding the patient, made this caution the more neceſſary.

In the beginning of the year 1618, he was ſent into France by king James, about ſome matters of importance; but being ſuſpected of a deſign to embroil affairs in that kingdom, he was commanded to leave it. In July 1624, he received the honour of knighthood from king James; and in Auguſt the ſame year he wrote a letter to his colleagues, the ordinary phyſicians of the king and prince, acquainting them, that as he was going to be abſent, probably for ſome time, from his duty at court, (with the permiſſion, however, of the king) he thought proper to ſelect for their peruſal certain forms of of prescription, and methods of practice, of which his experience had taught him the efficacy in the disorders to which his illustrious patients were most liable. Certain prudential rules for their conduct are prefixed, which shew the man of sense and liberal sentiments, but might perhaps be thought somewhat assuming and officious by those to whom they were addressed. It does not appear where he went at this time, nor how long he was absent. On the accession of Charles I. he was appointed first physician to him and his queen, and rose still higher in authority and reputation during that reign. He appears to have been in great favour with queen Henrietta, as indeed he had been with her royal predecessor; and it may be thought that he made himself acceptable and necessary to these ladies, by condescending to matters rather beneath the dignity of his profession. Among the numerous prescriptions for them, which make the subject of a separate book in his works, we find a vast proportion relating to cosmetics of every kind, pastes, lotions, dentifrices, sweet bags, hair powders and the like; and directions concerning certain feminine ornamental

mental minutiæ, rather deſerving the attention of the *friſeur* or corn-cutter than the phyſician. How far court phyſicians of every nation may be obliged to enter into theſe niceties, I pretend not to determine; but I confeſs there appears to me in the character of Mayerne, however reſpectable for knowledge and integrity, that ſpirit of inſinuating into favour by minute attentions, and of engroſſing every branch of medical truſt, which often diſtinguiſhes the phyſicians of other countries from the more generous and liberal ones of our own.

THE life of Mayerne, ſpent uniformly in the practice of his profeſſion at court and among the great, affords few anecdotes for the biographer. We find it mentioned by himſelf that in 1628 he was for ſome time abſent from his duty on account of a very ſevere illneſs with which his wife was attacked. In 1632 an inſtance of the eſteem in which he was held by the College of Phyſicians appears, in his being deſired to draw up their opinion concerning a perſon ſuſpected to have been poiſoned, which, from ſome difficulties that occurred on the trial, was required of them by his majesty. In this paper his name is signed next to that of the president. In 1635 he wrote a letter to the president of the College, complaining of one Evans, a minister and empiric, who had abused his name concerning the antimonial cup. The complaint was attended to; but the man's use of Mayerne's name, though falsely, is an evidence that he was considered as a patron and promoter of chemical medicine.

WE do not hear how he disposed of himself during the civil commotions which raged in the latter part of his life. He doubtless adhered to the royal party; for he was appointed nominal first physician to Charles II. after the decease of his father. Thus he enenjoyed the almost unparalleled honour of serving four kings successively in his medical capacity. At length, full of years, wealth, and reputation, he died at Chelsea in the eighty-second year of his age, March 15,* 1655. It is said that the immediate cause of

* ABOUT the 26th of March. *Wood Fast. Oxon. I.* 175.

his

his death proceeded from the effects of bad wine, and that he foretold the event to some friends with whom he had been drinking moderately at a tavern in the Strand. He was buried in the church of St. Martin's in the Fields, where the bodies of his mother, first wife, and five of his children had been deposited; and his funeral sermon was preached by a presbyterian minister. He left behind him an only daughter, who was married to the marquis de Montpouvillon. He bequeathed his library to the College of Physicians.

FROM a print extant of Sir Theodore Mayerne, he appears to have been very corpulent, with an open dignified countenance. He is said to have had this singularity, that he kept no regular meals, but had his table constantly covered, so that he could eat whenever he found himself disposed.

BESIDES the title of knighthood conferred upon him by Charles I. he was baron of Aulbone in France; but whether this was conferred or hereditary, I am not able to determine.

The only work which Sir Theod. Mayerne is ſaid to have publiſhed in his life time, was the apology before-mentioned, entitled *Apologia, in qua videre eſt, inviolatis Hippocratis & Galeni legibus, Remedia Chemicé præparata tuto uſurpari poſſe. Rupel.* 1603. Guy Patin, who was no friend to our author, attributes this piece to Seguin and Akakia the younger. Whether from the effect of this piece, or the ſucceſsful practice of Mayerne and the other patrons of chemical remedies, it is ſaid that the faculty of Paris ſoon retracted their cenſures, and extolled the writings and medicines of the chemiſts with as much ardour as they had before condemned them.

Of the other pieces which have been at different times publiſhed under the name of Mayerne, the following liſt is given.

Medicinal Counſels and Advices; and a *Treatiſe on the Gout*, written in French, and tranſlated into Latin and publiſhed by Theophilus Bonetus. This work was tranſlated into Engliſh by Dr. Thomas Sherley, phyſician in ordinary to Charles II. and publiſhed in 1676. 12mo. The author attributes the gout to the corroſive rofive quality of a certain *tartarous* matter, or *falt*, feparated from the mafs of blood, and thrown upon thofe parts which are moft apt to receive it. After fome directions for a regimen to prevent attacks of the gout, he proceeds to medicines, of which vomits and purgatives are the principal. The vomit which he principally approves, is antimonial wine, made by an infufion of crocus metallorum. To thofe who do not like medicines, he recommends the beaftly practice of gorging the ftomach once a month with a great quantity of food and drink, in order to provoke vomiting. Of purgatives, he beftows particular praifes on calomel, given to the dofe of a fcruple. Among the medicines which fweeten and correct the humours, he mentions *fugar of lead*, which he fays may be fafely taken inwardly with proper conferves. He gives a gout powder, one of the ingredients of which is *rafpings of a human fkull unburied*; and again, fpeaking of the good effects of abforbents, he particularly recommends *human bones* of the fame kind with the parts affected. Thefe tokens of fuperftition are not invalidated by a recipe contained in the fame book, of an unguent for hypochondriacal perſons, which he calls his *balſam of bats*. In the compoſition of this there enter, adders, bats, ſucking whelps, earth-worms, hog's greaſe, the marrow of a ſtag, and of the thigh-bone of an ox—ingredients fitter for the witches' cauldron in Macbeth, than a learned phyſician's preſcription. On the whole, this publication does not inſpire a very high idea of its celebrated author.

Praxeos Mayernianæ in morbis internis gravioribus & chronicis Syntagma; firſt publiſhed at London in 1690, by his godſon Sir Theodore de Vaux; who likewiſe in 1687 communicated to the Royal Society, *Mayerne's Account of the Diſeaſes of Dogs, with ſeveral Receipts for Canine Madneſs*, printed in the Philſophical Tranſactions of that year. The *Praxis Mayerniana* is a view of the method of cure uſed by this phyſician in a number of diſorders. It conſiſts almoſt entirely of preſcriptions, containing ſcarcely any thing of the deſcription of diſeaſes, or diſcrimination of their ſeveral ſtages and variations; and therefore will be thought of much leſs utility

utility than Dr. Charleton in his pompous preface ſeems to promiſe. The medicines preſcribed are numerous and extremely compound. Veſtiges of antient ſuperſtition frequently appear. The ſecundines of a woman at her firſt labour who has been delivered of a male child, the bowels of a mole cut open alive, mummy made of the lungs of a man who has ſuffered a violent death, the liver of frogs, and the blood of weaſels, are articles of his *materia medica*. Amulets of various kinds, ſimple and compound, are likewiſe directed. In one reſpect, however, the author's credulity ſeems in ſome degree regulated by good ſenſe. He was conſulted about a woman ſuſpected to be a demoniac. In his anſwer, he ſays, that though he does not doubt of the power of the devil in exciting diſturbances in the human body, he is likewiſe aware of the artifices of men: and that therefore he acknowledges only two certain marks of real poſſeſſion; one, where illiterate perſons become able to diſcourſe ſolidly and readily in various languages and on topics of different arts and ſciences; the other, where their bodies are taken up and ſuſpended for a

 conſidera-

considerable time in the air. If these criteria had been always applied, the number of demoniacs upon record would have been much lessened.

THERE are some particular observations in this book worthy of being noted. Under the head of epilepsy, the author mentions having met with a case, in which an epileptic person falling into an intermitting fever was entirely cured, after a few paroxysms, of his former disorder. Speaking of the cataract, he describes a singular operation performed by a female English oculist, which was, opening the cornea above the pupil with a needle, and discharging the aqueous humour, the foulness of which had obstructed vision. The operation was successful, the eye soon filling again, and the wound healing without a scar. Concerning vomitings, a curious story is related, of a woman's drinking by mistake a pint of antimonial wine in an apothecary's shop. When from its operation she was nearly expiring, the apothecary luckily gave her some cream of tartar, the first thing that came to hand; three or four drams of which instantly stopt the vomiting. It appears from this

this author that a mineral water at Wellinborough in Northamptonſhire was at that time in high repute. According to him, it contained a good deal of iron, ſome vitriol, and alum, or nitre. The formulæ of ſome noſtrums of Mayerne's are added at the end of this work. Several of them are preparations of iron and of mercury.

Tractatus de cura Gravidarum, added to an edition of the *Praxis Mayern.*

Epiſtol. de Gonorrheæ inveteratæ, & Carunculæ & Ulceris in meatu urinario curatione ad Georg. Mat. Koningium.

The ſubſtance of moſt of theſe articles is included in Dr. Joſeph Browne's publication, entitled *Mayernii Opera Medica, complectentia Conſilia, Epiſtolas & Obſervationes; Pharmacopœiam variaſque Medicamentorum formulas.* Lond. 1701. fol. In the preface, Dr. Browne complains that Dr. Charleton oppoſed the deſign of reprinting Mayerne's works entire, and would have had them abridged and methodized, and ſuch parts left out as greatly differed from modern practice. Browne did not

not agree to this opinion, but has publiſhed them in the order and form in which they were written, from M. S. S. lodged in the College of Phyſicians. The printing is extremely incorrect. The firſt book in this volume conſiſts of medical caſes treated by the author, to moſt of which the names of the patients are prefixed, who are, in general, perſons of the firſt quality in France and England. They comprehend a ſeries from 1605 to 1640. The deſcriptions are generally diſtinct, minute and judicious, and the reaſonings, though commonly founded upon the erroneous doctrines of that time, are yet acute and learned. The method of cure likewiſe for the moſt part appears founded upon rational principles and juſt obſervation; but the vaſt farrago of medicines preſcribed, the ſucceſſive effects of which are ſeldom related, confound one's ideas, and prevent thoſe practical concluſions which might otherwiſe be deduced from real caſes ſo circumſtantially drawn up. Notwithſtanding his ſuppoſed attachment to chemical remedies, not many of theſe occur among his preſcriptions, which are moſtly of the compound form of the Galenical

Galenical ſchool. Chalybeates and preparations from tartar are indeed pretty frequently met with, but mercurials and antimonials ſcarcely ever. The great proportion of hypochondriac and hyſteric caſes, in both ſexes, may appear ſomewhat remarkable, and contradictory to the ſuppoſition that the frequency of theſe diſorders is a modern variation in the ſtate of diſeaſes. But it muſt be remembered, that almoſt all Mayerne's patients were people of rank. We have already mentioned the caſe of prince Henry as one of the moſt important. It affords a complete ſpecimen of the practice in a putrid fever before the uſe of Peruvian bark; which might in all probability have been given here with much advantage, as there was a fair intermiſſion of the fever at the beginning. Purgatives, cooling cordials, and the ſuppoſed alexipharmicks, ſuch as bezoar, &c. were exhibited; and as the laſt reſource, diaſcordium, without which no one could then die *ſecundum artem*, was adminiſtered. A ſpontaneous bleeding at the noſe ſeemed to Dr. Mayerne an indication for veneſection, which after much oppoſition was performed on the eighth

eighth day of the diſeaſe. The blood was of a broken diſſolved texture; and notwithſtanding the temporary relief this operation ſeemed to afford, moſt practitioners at preſent would, I imagine, approve the conduct of the other phyſicians, who unanimouſly refuſed to allow its repetition, although it was much preſſed by Mayerne. The caſe of the celebrated Iſaac Caſaubon likewiſe deſerves notice. This learned man was ſeized with a gradual difficulty, and at length a total ſuppreſſion of urine, of which he died in great torture. On diſſection, there appeared to be a total obliteration of the canal of the urethra, owing to a kind of ſac communicating with the bladder which received all the urine. A caſe in which caruncles and ſtrictures in the urethra were complicated with a ſtone in the bladder, gives room for the author to exhibit much knowledge of ſurgery in the treatment. The uſe of bougies, both ſimple and medicated, is very exactly and judiciouſly directed; and a gangrene which ſupervened after lithotomy is managed with much ſkill. Indeed, he left behind him ſeveral writings expreſsly upon chirurgical ſubjects, which Dr. Browne had a deſign a deſign of publiſhing, but it miſcarried for want of encouragement.

THE ſecond part of this volume conſiſts of a Pharmacopœia, in which a great number of formulæ, moſtly collected from other authors, are thrown together with very little order or method. They are both Chemical and Galenical; and the former are in much greater number and variety than thoſe which are mentioned in his own private practice. The exuberance of chalybeate preparations ſhows him to have been fond of that remedy; and this is confirmed by a Latin advertiſement prefixed to the book concerning the ſale of Dr. Mayerne's chalybeate pills. Little of neatneſs and elegance can be expected in the formulæ of that day; and this part of the work is rather curious than uſeful. The folly of amulets, ſympathetic ointments, and antidotes was not yet quite exploded; and the preſcriptions for analeptics and provocatives to be met with in this collection, muſt be conſidered as ſtill more derogatory from the dignity of the profeſſion, than the coſmetic branch of court practice which we before took occaſion

occaſion to cenſure.* They are however a kind of progreſſion towards another part of our phyſician's character, that of a cook; for to him is attributed a book entitled *Excellent and well-approved Receipts and Experiments in Cookery, with the beſt Way of Preſerving*, &c. printed in 1658.

HE appears in a much more reſpectable light as employing his knowledge in chemiſtry to the advancement of the fine arts. We are told in the life of Petitot the famous painter in enamel, † that this artiſt perfected his ſkill in colouring by his viſit to England, where he became acquainted with Sir Theodore Mayerne, then firſt phyſician to Charles I. who had by a courſe of experiments diſcovered the principal colours to be uſed for enamel, and the proper means of vitrifying them. Mayerne introduced this artiſt to the king, who went often to ſee him work, as he took pleaſure in painting and in chemical experiments, to which his phyſician had given him a turn.

* THERE is a deſcription as groſs and laſcivious as any thing in old John of Gaddeſden, in Prax. Mayern. p. 407.

† Brit. Biogr. tom. VI. p. 139.

NATURAL

Natural philoſophy was another branch of ſcience which he appears to have cultivated. He was the editor of Mouffet's poſthumous work on inſects; in an epiſtle prefixed to which, he recites, in a manner that ſhews him well acquainted with the ſubject, many of the wonders obſervable in this minute claſs of animals.

ROBERT FLUDD,

OR, as he ſtiled himſelf in Latin, *De Fluctibus*, ſecond ſon of Sir Thomas Fludd, treaſurer of war to queen Elizabeth, was born in 1574 at Milgate in Kent. He was educated at St. John's College, Oxford; and after taking his degree in arts, attached himſelf to the ſtudy of phyſic, and ſpent almoſt ſix years in his travels through the principal countries of Europe. It was probably during theſe peregrinations that he imbibed a taſte for the Roſycrucian philoſophy, of which he ever after was a moſt ſtrenuous ſupporter, and indeed almoſt the only one who became eminent

nent in it in this kingdom. He proceeded as doctor of physic in 1605, and about that time settled in London, and was made a fellow of the College of Physicians. He was a very voluminous author in his sect, diving into the farthest profundities and most mysterious obscurities of the Rosie-cross, and blending in a most extraordinary manner divinity, chemistry, natural philosophy, and metaphysics. Such a vein of warm enthusiasm runs through his works, that we may readily suppose him to have been a believer in the mystical jargon of his system. He is said to have used a kind of sublime unintelligible cant to his patients, which by inspiring them with greater faith in his skill, might in some cases contribute to their cure. There is no doubt, at least, that it would assist his reputation; and accordingly we find that he was eminent in his medical capacity. His philosophy, however, whether owing to the dawning of a more enlightened period, in this island, or a less natural taste for such abstruse speculations in his countrymen, was received with less applause at home than abroad. The celebrated Gassendus had a controversy with him; which

which ſhows, at leaſt, that he was not conſidered as an inſignificant writer. As the Roſycrucian ſect is now entirely extinct, I ſhall not trouble the reader with the long liſt of his works, given by Wood. They are moſtly written in Latin, and the largeſt of them, entitled *Nexus utriuſque Coſmi, &c.* has ſome extremely ſingular prints in it, which are only to be underſtood by a ſecond-ſighted adept.*

Dr. Fludd died at his houſe in Coleman-ſtreet, London, on September 8, 1637, and was buried in the pariſh church of his native place.

It is ſaid that Dr. Fludd was in poſſeſſion of the M. S. S. of Simon Forman, the aſtrologer. This circumſtance leads me to ſay ſomething of the pretenders to phyſic and aſtrology, who were much in vogue about that time, and continued to be held in ſome eſtimation till the beginning of the preſent century. We have ſeen that the ſtudies of mathematics, aſtronomy and medicine were

* Granger, *Biograph. Hiſt.*

early united in ſeveral perſons who have been the ſubjects of theſe memoirs. Real aſtronomy gave birth to judicial aſtrology; which offering an ample field to enthuſiaſm and impoſture, was eagerly purſued by many who had no ſcientific purpoſe in view. It was connected with various juggling tricks and deceptions, affected an obſcure jargon of language, and inſinuated itſelf into every thing in which the hopes and fears of mankind were concerned. The profeſſors of this pretended ſcience were generally perſons of mean education, in whom low cunning ſupplied the place of real knowledge. Moſt of them engaged in the empirical practice of phyſic, and ſome, through the credulity of the times, even arrived at a degree of eminence in it; yet ſince the whole foundation of their art was folly and deceit, I cannot think them proper ſubjects for a more particular relation. Chemical empirics, although enthuſiaſtical, and perhaps in general ignorant, may introduce valuable improvements in the practice of medicine: but aſtrological impoſtors never can. I ſhall therefore take no farther notice of this ſect; but refer the curious

curious reader to *Lilly's Account of his own Life*, in which he has characterized many of the moſt noted amongſt them, as well as himſelf, in ſuch a manner as can leave no doubt of their united ignorance and knavery.

THOMAS WINSTON,

BORN in 1575, was the ſon of a carpenter, the place of whoſe abode we are not informed of. He was educated in Clare hall, Cambridge, of which he became fellow. In 1602 he took the degree of M. A. and then went abroad for improvement in the ſtudy of phyſic. He attended the lectures of Fabricius ab Aquapendente and Proſper Alpinus at Padua, and of Caſpar Bauhine at Baſil, and took the degree of doctor at Padua. On his return to England, he graduated again at Cambridge in 1607. He afterwards ſettled in London, where he became eminent in his profeſſion; and in 1613 was admitted a candidate of the

College of Physicians, and the next year was made fellow.

On the death of Dr. Mounsell, professor of physic in Gresham college, Dr. Winston was chosen on the 25th of October 1615, to succeed him. One of his competitors was Dr. Simeon Fox, son of the celebrated martyrologist; of whom, and Dr. Argent, it is recorded, that they were the last presidents of the College of Physicians who used to ride on horseback in London to visit their patients. Dr. Winston held his professorship till the year 1642, during which time he acquired a handsome fortune; but then, upon permission of the House of Lords, he went over to France on a sudden, without having settled his affairs, or provided for the security of his estate. The cause of this hasty departure seems to have been some apprehensions from the parliament, whose party then began to prevail, and whom he had probably offended by the discovery of some secrets entrusted to him. Dr. Hamey, in his M. S. life of Dr. Winston, says he withdrew himself *præ metu Angeronæ** *sæpius læsæ*,

* The Goddess of Silence.

& jam

& jam pœnas minitantis. His profeſſorſhip in Greſham college thus becoming vacant, after he had been ſix months abſent, Dr. Paul De Laune was choſen in his room.

He ſtaid abroad about ten years; and in 1652, having, by the intereſt of his friends, accommodated matters with the perſons in power, he returned to England, and was reſtored to his profeſſorſhip, and what elſe he poſſeſſed at the time of his departure. Of this affair, Whitelocke, in his Memoirs, gives the following account. "July 10, 1652. Dr. "Winſton, a phyſician, in the beginning of "the late troubles, by leave of the Houſe of "Lords went over into France, and there "continued till very lately, that he returned "into England. In his abſence, none being "here to look after his buſineſs for him, his "eſtate was ſequeſtered, as if he had been a "delinquent; and his place and lodgings of "phyſic profeſſor in Greſham college were "taken from him: though he had never "acted any thing againſt the parliament, but "had been out of England all the time of "the troubles. Whereupon application being "made to the committee of ſequeſtrations, an "order was procured for his being reſtored to "his place and lodgings in Greſham college; "and the ſequeſtration of his eſtate, which "was £500 *per ann.* was alſo taken off." From the expreſſion "had never acted any thing againſt the parliament," it would ſeem, as profeſſor Ward obſerves,* that his offence had conſiſted in words only, not in actions. At the time of his leaving the kingdom, he was one of the elects of the College of Phyſicians; and this place being alſo forfeited by his abſence, he was re-choſen on a vacancy in June 1653.

He did not long enjoy this favourable change in his circumſtances, for he died October 24, 1655, being then eighty years of age.

He was much valued as a gentleman and a ſcholar, as well as an eminent phyſician. Meric Caſaubon calls him "the great ornament of his profeſſion." Dr. Hamey's praiſe will ſcarcely be thought very advantageous to

* *Lives of Greſham Profeſſors*; from which this article is extracted.

his

his character. He commends him for supporting the dignity of the faculty againſt the apothecaries, making uſe of but one himſelf, whom he commanded like a maſter; "*heriliter imperavit.*" On this account he eſteems him a benefactor to the College. The members of that learned body at preſent, ſeem to think they can ſuſtain the dignity of their profeſſion, without putting on the manners of a baſhaw.

Dr. Winston did not publiſh any thing; but after his death a treatiſe appeared, entitled

Anatomy Lectures at Greſham College: By that eminent and learned Phyſician, Dr. Thomas Winſton. Lond. 1659, 1664. 8vo.

The editor, in an epiſtle prefixed, ſuppoſes, from certain expreſſions, that they were alſo read by the author in his appointed courſe at the College of Phyſicians. They comprehend an entire body of anatomy, with the improvements down to his time, which includes the diſcoveries of Harvey; and were ſuppoſed the moſt complete and accurate then extant in the Engliſh language.

TOBIAS VENNER

WAS born of genteel parents at Petherton, near Bridgewater, in Somersetshire, in the year 1577, and at the age of seventeen became a commoner of St. Alban's hall, Oxford. After taking a degree in arts, he entered upon the physic line, and practised for a time about Oxford. In 1613, he took the degree of doctor; and returning to his own country, practised for many years at Bridgewater; but afterwards, at or near Bath. He was highly esteemed in that part of the country for skill in his profession, and maintained the character of an upright and charitable person. He died March 27, 1660; and was buried in St. Peter's church in Bath, where a monument with a large inscription, by Dr. Pierce of that city, was erected to his memory.

Dr. Venner acquired great popular fame by a work of his, entitled "*Via Recta* "*ad Vitam longam*: or A plain Philoso- "phical Demonstration of the Nature, Facul- "ties

" ties and Effects of all such Things as by Way " of Nourishments make for the Preservation " of Health, with divers necessary dietetical " Observations; as also of the true Use and " Effects of Sleep, Exercise, Excretions, and " Perturbations, with just Applications to " every Age, Constitution of Body, and Time " of Year." This copious title will sufficiently acquaint the reader with the subject of the work. It was published in two separate parts; the first in 1620, and the second in 1623: and both were incorporated in subsequent editions. It is a plain practical piece; extremely different in manner from Dr. Moufet's *Treatise on Foods*, though similar in subject. His account of the several articles treated of, is compiled (though without any quotations) from the current authors of that time; and his rules and admonitions, delivered with all due gravity and authority, are equally trite. His style and manner are well calculated for a popular work, being plain, grave and diffuse. Dr. Guidott, in his *Lives of Bath Physicians*, attempting to ridicule the good doctor, quotes from him this memorable observation, that " a gammon of bacon

" is

"is of the ſame nature with the reſt of "the hog."*

To the edition of the *Via Recta* in 1638, were added the following pieces.

A Compendious Treatiſe concerning the Nature, Uſe and Efficacy of the Bathes at Bath. Dedicated to the queen. This is a very ſhort piece, conſiſting chiefly of general directions concerning the uſe of the waters, every where referring the patient to the advice of a *phyſician reſident in the place* for particulars. It is dubious, from his language, whether the waters were uſed internally in his time. He no where even hints that they were; on the contrary, all his directions reſpect bathing: yet his liſt of diſeaſes for which Bath offers a remedy, includes ſome which would ſeem to require drinking rather than bathing; as ſome windy and hydropic diſorders, tumours of the ſpleen and liver, and the jaundice.

Advertiſement concerning the taking of Phyſic in the Spring. This is a very trifling little piece,

* He ſays it is of the ſame nature, but not ſo good; being harder of digeſtion.

piece, chiefly confifting of invective againft empirics.

Cenfure concerning the Water of St. Vincent's Rocks near Briftol. This is faid to be the firft treatife relating to Briftol water. It contains plain directions for its ufe, particularly in cafes of ftone and ulcers of the bladder, for which it was then much celebrated.

Brief and accurate Treatife concerning the taking of the Fume of Tobacco. This is a tolerably fenfible account of the properties of tobacco, in which he attempts to reftrict its ufe to medical purpofes, and to reftrain the promifcuous cuftom of taking it, which was then become extremely fafhionable.

WILLIAM HARVEY.

ALTHOUGH many of the perfons we have hitherto commemorated were eminent in various branches of literature, and either adorned their profeffion by elegant accom-

accomplishments, or enriched their art by useful observations; yet none of them can be considered as giving a new æra to the medical science in general, by great and signal discoveries. The barrenness of our biographical records in this respect, is however amply repaid by the renowned subject of the present article; who enlightened the world with the investigation of a law in the animal œconomy, of such fundamental importance, as justly to place his name in the highest rank of natural philosophers. The same services which Newton afterwards rendered to optics and astronomy by his theories of light and gravitation, Harvey rendered to anatomy by his true doctrine of the circulation: and from the intimate connection of this science with the healing art, the practical utility of this discovery has not been inferior to its speculative beauty; insomuch that Sir Thomas Browne might with some reason prefer it to the discovery of the new world.

William Harvey was descended from a respectable family in the county of Kent. His father, Thomas Harvey, had seven sons and

and two daughters. Five of the ſons were brought up to a commercial life, and engaged in the Turkey trade, by which they acquired plentiful fortunes. William, the eldeſt ſon, who happily for mankind, choſe a literary profeſſion, was born at Folkſtone, in Kent, on the firſt of April, 1578. At ten years of age he was ſent to the grammar ſchool in Canterbury; and having here laid a proper foundation of claſſical learning, he was removed to Gonvile and Caius college in Cambridge, and admitted there as a penſioner in May 1593. After ſpending ſix years at this univerſity in thoſe academical ſtudies which are preparatory to a learned profeſſion, he went abroad for the acquiſition of medical knowledge; and travelling through France and Germany, he fixed himſelf at Padua. The univerſity of this city was then in the height of its reputation for the ſtudy of phyſic; for which it was principally indebted to Fabricius ab Aquapendente, the profeſſor of anatomy, whoſe lectures Harvey attended with the utmoſt diligence; as he did likewiſe thoſe of Minadous in the practice of medicine, and Caſſerius in ſurgery. Here he took his doctor's tor's degree, the diploma for which, drawn up in extraordinary terms of approbation,* is dated April 25, 1602, when Harvey had just completed his twenty-fourth year.

In the course of the same year he returned to his own country; and after having again graduated at Cambridge, he settled in the practice of his profession at London. At the age of twenty-six he married the daughter of Launcelot Browne, M. D. by whom he never had any children. How long she lived with him we are not informed; but from a bequest in the will of John Harvey, the doctor's brother, it appears that she was living in 1645.

In 1604 he was admitted a candidate of the College of Physicians, and was elected fellow

* In quo quidem examine adeo mirifice & excellentissime se gessit, talemque ac tantam ingenii, memoriæ, & doctrinæ vim ostendit, ut expectatione quam de se apud omnes concitaverat, longissime superata, a prædictis Exc^{mis}. Doctoribus unanimiter & concorditer, cunctisque suffragiis, ac eorum nemine penitus atque penitus discrepante, aut dissentiente, nec hæsitante quidem, idoneus & sufficientissimus in Artibus & Medicina fuerit judicatus.

Diploma, *printed in the College Edition of Harvey's Works.*

about

about three years after. About this time the governors of St. Bartholomew's hoſpital made an order, that on the deceaſe of Dr. Wilkinſon, phyſician to that charity, Dr. Harvey ſhould ſuceeed him in his office; which event took place the next year. A more important circumſtance in the life of this great man occurred in the year 1615, when the College of Phyſicians appointed him reader of the anatomical and chirurgical lectures founded by Lord Lumley and Dr. Caldwall. It was in the courſe of theſe lectures, that he firſt publicly delivered his new doctrines concerning the circulation; as ſufficiently appears from ſome M. S. S. of his, ſtill extant, in which the principal propoſitions concerning that important fact are laid down; and likewiſe from his referring to the lectures in the dedication of his book to the College of Phyſicians. The index of his M. S. *De Anatomia Univerſa*, preſerved in the Britiſh Muſeum, which contains theſe propoſitions, is dated as early as April 16, 17, 18; 1616; but the year 1619 is uſually ſuppoſed the time of his firſt openly diſcloſing his opinions on the ſubject. That this great diſcovery was firſt

firſt made public in an anatomical ſchool at London, is certainly a very honourable circumſtance in the literary hiſtory of that metropolis; which, however celebrated as the ſeat of opulence and ſplendour, has not been in general conſidered as a nurſery of ſcience.

THE character of Harvey now began to recommend him to the notiee of the court, and he was appointed phyſician to king James I. though in what preciſe year we are not able to aſcertain. From a letter of the king to Harvey, dated February 3, 1623, it appears, that he had been for ſome time phyſician extraordinary to his majeſty; who, as a mark of ſingular favour, grants him permiſſion to conſult with the ordinary phyſicians concerning his health, and promiſes to conſtitute him one of that number on the firſt vacancy; which, however, did not take place till ſeven years after, in the next reign. In the year 1627, he was appointed one of the elects of the College of Phyſicians; and in 1628, his doctrine of the circulation, which had been gradually maturating for ſeveral years, during a ſeries of patient experiment and cautious reaſon-

reaſoning, was firſt committed to the preſs at Frankfort. The choice of this city for the place of publication is ſuppoſed to have ariſen from its celebrated fairs, by means of which, books printed there were rapidly circulated throughout all Germany, and the greateſt part of Europe. The great commotions this work excited in the learned world, the attempts of ſome to refute his arguments, and of others to rob him of the honour of original diſcovery, will be more properly diſplayed when we come to the ſeparate conſideration of his literary character. I ſhall now only obſerve, that notwithſtanding the rank he held in his profeſſion, and the favourable reception of his opinions by his brethren of the faculty at home, ſuch is the general prejudice againſt an innovator, that we find him complaining to a friend, that his practice conſiderably declined after the publication of of his book.

For this mortification he was, however, greatly recompenſed by the regard and favour of his royal maſter Charles I. whoſe attachment to the arts and ſciences formed a conſpicuous part of his character. It is not without a degree of pardonable vanity that Harvey deſcribes this king, with ſome of the nobleſt perſons about his court, as deigning to be the ſpectators and witneſſes of his experiments. The intereſt his majeſty took in the ſucceſs of his anatomical reſearches was of ſingular ſervice to him in his enquiries concerning the nature of generation, as the king's favourite diverſion of ſtag-hunting furniſhed him with the oportunity of diſſecting a vaſt number of animals of that ſpecies in a pregnant ſtate. A farther mark of Charles's eſteem of the man, as well as of the phyſician, appears in his appointing Harvey to accompany the young duke of Lenox in his travels; on which occaſion, the governors of St. Bartholomew's hoſpital allowed him to delegate his office to Dr. Smyth during his abſence. Some years after, Harvey, by his influence, cauſed ſeveral regulations to paſs for the correction of various abuſes which had crept into the hoſpital, particularly reſpecting the reception and management of patients, and the intruſion of the ſurgeons into the phyſician's department. About the ſame time,

as

as his office at court obliged him to a cloſe attendance upon the king's perſon, the governors appointed Dr. Andrews his aſſiſtant in the hoſpital, yet ſtill, in conſideration of his merit and ſervices, continued his former ſalary. He viſited Scotland, probably in attendance on the king, during this period; and has given a ſpecimen of his obſervations there, in a moſt elegant and picturesque deſcription of the Baſs iſland.

The civil wars now breaking out, Harvey, who was attached to the king by office, gratitude and affection, accompanied him in his ſeveral journeys; and after the battle of Edge-hill he went, with the reſt of the royal houſehold, to Oxford. Here he was incorporated doctor of phyſic, on December 7, 1642; and in 1645, by his majeſty's mandate, he was made warden of Merton college, in the room of Dr. Nathaniel Brent, who, in compliance with the prevailing party, had left the univerſity and taken the covenant. This preferment was merited by Harvey, not only on account of his fidelity and ſervices, but his ſufferings in the royal cauſe: for, during the confusions of the times, his house in London was plundered of the furniture, and, what was a much heavier loss, of his papers, containing a great number of anatomical observations, particularly with regard to the generation of insects. This was an irretrievable injury, and has extorted from him the following pathetic, but gentle complaint. "Atque hæc dum agimus, ignoscant mihi niveæ animæ, si, summarum "injuriarum memor, levem gemitum effudero. Doloris mihi hæc causa est: cum "inter nuperos nostros tumultus, & bella "plusquam civilia, serenissimum regem, "idque non solum Senatus permissione, sed "& jussu, sequor; rapaces quædam manus, "non modo ædium mearum supellectilem "omnem expilarunt; sed etiam, quæ mihi "causa gravior querimoniæ, adversaria mea, "multorum annorum laboribus parta, e mu"seo meo summanarunt. Quo factum est, "ut observationes plurimæ, præsertim de "generatione insectorum, cum reipublicæ "literariæ, ausim dicere, detrimento, pe"rierint." *

* *Exercitat.* LXVIII. ad finem.

HE

He did not long poſſeſs the maſterſhip of Merton college; for, upon the ſurrender of Oxford to the parliament, he left the place and went to London, and Dr. Brent ſoon after reſumed his office. From this time he ſeems to have lived in a retired manner, reſiding either at London, at Lambeth, or in the houſe of one of his brothers at Richmond. In 1651, the ſeventy-firſt year of his age, he was prevailed upon by his intimate friend Dr. George Ent, to publiſh, or rather to ſuffer him to publiſh, his other great work, his *Exercitations on the Generation of Animals*, which had employed ſo large a portion of his time and attention. Dr. Ent, in his prefatory epiſtle to the College of Phyſicians, gives a very elegant and pleaſing account of his interview with Harvey on this occaſion. I found him, ſays he, in his retirement not far from town, with a ſprightly and chearful countenance, inveſtigating, like Democritus, the nature of things. Aſking if all was well with him, "how can that be," he replied, "when the "ſtate is ſo agitated with ſtorms, and I myſelf "am yet in the open ſea? And indeed," added he, "were not my mind ſolaced by "my studies, and the recollection of the observations I have formerly made, there is "nothing which should make me desirous of "a longer continuance. But thus employed, "this obscure life, and vacation from public "cares, which disquiets other minds, is the "medicine of mine." He goes on to relate a philosophical conversation between them, that brought on the mention of these papers of his, which the public had so long expected. After some modest altercation, Harvey brought them all to him, with permission, either to publish them immediately, or to suppress them till some future time. I went from him, says Dr. Ent, like another Jason, in possession of the golden fleece; and when I came home, and perused the pieces singly, I was amazed that so vast a treasure should have been so long hidden; and that while others with great parade exhibit to the public their stale trash, this person should seem to make so little account of his admirable observations. Indeed, no one appears to have possessed in a greater degree that genuine modesty which distinguishes the real philosopher from the superficial pretender to science. His great discovery difcovery was not publicly offered to the world, till after a nine years' probation among his colleagues at home; and the labours of all the latter part of his life would fcarcely have appeared till after his death, had not the importunities of a friend extorted them from him.

In December 1652, the College of Phyficians teftified their regard for their illuftrious affociate in a manner fingularly honourable. They voted the erection of his ftatue in their hall, with the following infcription,

GULIELMO HARVEIO
VIRO MONUMENTIS SUIS IMMORTALI
HOC INSUPER COLLEGIUM MEDICORUM LONDINENSE
POSUIT
QUI ENIM SANGUINIS MOTUM
UT ET
ANIMALIBUS ORTUM DEDIT MERUIT ESSE
STATOR PERPETUUS.

This obligation foon met with a fuitable return. On the fecond of February following, Harvey, inviting the members to a fplendid entertainment, prefented the College with the deed of gift of an elegantly furnifhed convocation-room, and a muſeum filled with choice books and chirurgical inſtruments, which he had built at his own expence in their garden.

In 1654, on the reſignation of the preſidency by Dr. Prujean, the College appointed Harvey, in his abſence, to ſucceed him; and proroguing the meeting to the next day, deputed two of the elects to acquaint him with this reſolution. Harvey then came, and in a handſome ſpeech returned them thanks for the honour they had done him, but declined the office on account of his age and infirmities; at the ſame time recommending the re-election of Dr. Prujean, which was unanimouſly complied with. He ſtill however frequented the meetings of the College; and his attachment to that body was ſhewn yet more conſpicuouſly in 1656, when, at the firſt anniverſary feaſt inſtituted by himſelf, he gave up his paternal eſtate of £56 *per ann.* in perpetuity, to their uſe. The particular purpoſes of this donation were, the inſtitution of an annual feaſt, at which a Latin oration ſhould be ſpoken in commemoration of the benefactors of the College; a gratuity for the orator; and a proviſion for the

the keeper of his library and muſeum. This attention to perpetuate a ſpirit of concord and ſocial friendſhip among his brethren muſt ſuggeſt an amiable idea of his benevolent and liberal ſentiments. At the ſame time he reſigned his office of lecturer, which he had till then diſcharged, to Dr. Scarborough.

He now with difficulty ſupported the burden of years and infirmities; and at length, on the third of June, 1658, having completed his eightieth year, he quietly ſunk under the load. Concerning the manner of his death, a nameleſs report was propagated, that unable to bear the increaſing calamities of old age, which were aggravated by the ſudden loſs of ſight, he put an end to his ſufferings by drinking poiſon. This ſtain on his memory will be beſt removed, by relating the particulars of his deceaſe, as given in an oration before the College, by Dr. Wilſon, a few days after the event. He laments that the uſual ſerenity of Harvey's temper was in his latter days clouded by numerous infirmities, and eſpecially by the excruciating pains of a ſevere gout: but alledges, that when drawing

drawing near his end, having compoſed his mind as to all his remaining concerns, he examined his pulſe, as if marking with a philoſophical attention the progreſs of approaching diſſolution; and thus, with the utmoſt tranquillity and reſignation, yielded up his breath. His body, a few days after his death, was removed in funeral proceſſion to Hempſted in Eſſex, all the Fellows of the College attending it to a conſiderable diſtance from the city. His remains were depoſited in a vault in the church of that place, where a monument was erected to his memory.

By his will he bequeathed the greateſt part of his effects to his brother Eliab Harvey, a merchant in London; his houſehold furniture among his relations; his books to the College of Phyſicians; legacies by way of memorial to his friends Drs. George Ent, and Charles Scarborough; gratuities to his ſervants; and £30 to St. Bartholomew's hoſpital. From this account it would ſeem that he did not die rich.

The private character of this great man appears to have been in every reſpect worthy of of his public reputation. Chearful, candid and upright, he was not the prey of any mean or ungentle paffion. He was as little difpofed by nature to detract from the merits of others, or make an oftentatious difplay of his own, as neceffitated to ufe fuch methods for advancing his fame. The many antagonifts whom his renown, and the novelty of his opinions excited, were, in general, treated by him with modeft and temperate language, frequently very different from their own; and while he refuted their arguments, he decorated them with all due praifes. He lived on terms of perfect harmony and friendfhip with his brethren of the College; and feems to have been very little ambitious of engroffing a difproportionate fhare of medical practice. In extreme old age, pain and ficknefs were faid to have rendered him fomewhat irritable in his temper; and as an inftance of want of command over himfelf at that feafon, it is related, that in the paroxyfms of the gout he could not be prevented from plunging the affected joint in cold water: but who can think it ftrange that when the body was almoft worn down, the mind fhould

alfo

alſo be debilitated? It is certain that the profoundeſt veneration for the great Cauſe of all thoſe wonders he was ſo well acquainted with, appears eminently conſpicuous in every part of his works. He was uſed to ſay, that he never diſſected the body of any animal, without diſcovering ſomething which he had not expected or conceived of, and in which he recognized the hand of an all-wiſe Creator. To His particular agency, and not to the operation of general laws, he aſcribed all the phænomena of nature. In familiar converſation, Harvey was eaſy and unaſſuming; and ſingularly clear in expreſſing his ideas. His mind was furniſhed with an ample ſtore of knowledge, not only in matters connected with his profeſſion, but in moſt of the objects of liberal enquiry, eſpecially in antient and modern hiſtory, and the ſcience of politics. He took great delight in reading the antient poets, Virgil in particular, with whoſe divine productions he is ſaid to have been ſometimes ſo tranſported, as to throw the book from him, with exclamations of rapture. To complete his character, he did not want that poliſh and courtly addreſs, which are neceſſary to the ſcholar who would alſo appear as a gentleman.

I SHALL

I SHALL now endeavour to give a concife, but diftinct account of what was done by this eminent perfon for the improvement of fcience; and in order to this, it will be neceffary firft, to take a general view of the progrefs which had been made by his predeceffors in thofe enquiries, which were the objects of his particular attention.

As far as we can underftand the confufed and contradictory language of the antient anatomifts concerning the fanguiferous fyftem, it feems to have been the opinion of the earlieft among them, that the veins, having their origin in the liver, were the only veffels carrying the blood through the body; that in thefe it moved backwards and forwards, with an irregular flux and reflux; and that the arteries, arifing from the heart, contained the animal fpirits, which were elaborated in that organ: that this was the cafe in a natural and healthy ftate; but that when the body was difeafed, the blood fometimes forced its way into the arteries. This fyftem is in part laid down by Hippocrates; but was principally maintained by Erafiftratus. Galen was the firft who made

made an approach to the true doctrine, by asserting, that the arteries always contained blood in the living animal; that much blood is also contained in the left ventricle of the heart; and even that a contraction of the arteries propels the blood into the veins: but, on the other hand, he always supposes that the blood flows from the right side of the heart into the vena cava, and thence through the body; that the arteries only receive blood from the veins; that the circulatory motion from one set of vessels to another is not constant; that all the blood which goes to the lungs is employed in their nutrition; and that the liver, rather than the heart, is the fountain of blood. He describes with accuracy the valves of the heart, but had no right conception of their action.

The opinions of Galen were of such inviolable authority for many centuries after, and experimental enquiries were so much neglected, that we need not wonder no advance was made in this important part of physiology till the time of Vesalius. This great man, who may be regarded as the father of modern anatomy,

anatomy, appears to have paid very particular attention to this ſubject. He confirms Galen's aſſertion, that the arteries always contain blood, by cutting out a piece of artery included between two ligatures. He next proves that there is a motion of the blood from the heart towards the extremities, through the arteries; and that this motion is rapid and violent; and obſerves that when the heart contracts, the arteries are filled. He remarks that when an artery is divided, the motion of the blood ceaſes below the diviſion, but is reſtored if a reed be inſerted into the divided ends; and alſo mentions, that when a ligature is made round a vein, the part neareſt the heart ſubſides. Yet, in contradiction to all this, he alſo ſuppoſes, with the antients, that the blood moves from the heart through the veins: ſo far could prejudice operate on a perſon who had thrown off its yoke to a greater degree than any one in his time; and had purſued, in its higheſt vigour, the true experimental method of enquiry.

A LITTLE before Veſalius publiſhed his works, and ſome time after, Servetus, a

Spaniſh phyſician, ſo well known by the cruel perſecution he underwent from Calvin, printed two theological tracts, in which he aſſerted the communication of the pulmonary artery and veins; that through them the blood paſſes from the right to the left ſide of the heart; and that the blood flows into the lungs not merely for the nutrition of that organ, but in order to be elaborated and ſubtilized, by the reception of a ſpirit from the air in inſpiration, and the exhalation of a fuliginous matter in expiration. This important part of the true ſyſtem was not, however, founded upon experiment, but was an ingenious hypotheſis, which its author would have found it difficult to ſupport, ſince he was ignorant of the force of the heart in propelling the blood, and the action of its valves in determining that force to a particular direction. In other points he adopted the errors of Galen; ſuppoſing the liver and veins to be the ſeat of the blood, and the heart and arteries that of the vital ſpirit, which was at times communicated to the blood by anaſtomoſes.

In 1569, Realdus Columbus, an excellent anatomiſt, publiſhed a book at Venice, in which

which he more particularly deſcribes the paſſage of the blood from the right to the left ſide of the heart, through the lungs; and alſo demonſtrates that the ſtructure of the ſigmoid valves at the beginning of the pulmonary artery muſt prevent the reflux of the blood into the heart; and that the tricuſpid valves muſt have the ſame effect in preventing the return of the blood received by the right ventricle from the *vena cava*. But he denies the muſcular ſtructure of the heart; gives no experiment to prove the communication between the pulmonary artery and veins; and makes the liver the fountain from whence the body is ſupplied with blood by means of the veins.

Cæsalpinus, who publiſhed about twelve years after, adopts a ſyſtem ſtill nearer the true one, though mixed with errors and inconſiſtencies. He ſuppoſes, after Ariſtotle, two kinds of blood, one ſerving for the increaſe of the body, the other for its aliment. The former he derives from the liver into the *vena cava*, whence he imagines it to be attracted by the heat of the heart into the right ventricle.

cle. Then, purſuing the reaſoning of Columbus concerning the valves of the heart, he traces the blood through the lungs (where he ſuppoſes it not to receive a ſpirituous nature from the air, but only to be cooled by it) to the left ventricle, and thence to the *aorta*, the valves of which prevent its return. He now conceives that the blood putting on a ſpirituous and alimentary nature, undergoes an effervefcence, which diſtends the heart and arteries; during which diſtention, the blood and vital ſpirits are carried through the arteries to all parts of the body; while at the ſame time the *auctive aliment* is by means of anaſtomoſes elicited from the veins. The heart and arteries then become flaccid till a new effervefcence is generated; and this alternation is the cauſe of the pulſe. Further, he alledges that the extreme ramifications of the arteries communicate with thoſe of the veins; and that *during ſleep* the blood with the vital ſpirit flows from the arteries to the veins; which he infers from the tumefaction of the veins, and diminution of the pulſe of the arteries, at that period. With reſpect to the tumefaction of a tied vein between the ligature and

and the extremities, after much labour to account for it, he at length offers as a reaſon, that when the veins are cloſed by a ligature, the blood flows back to its origin, leſt by its being intercepted, it ſhould be extinguiſhed. Thus it appears, that although Cæſalpinus admitted a circulation, he did not conceive of it as conſtant and rapid, nor was acquainted with its real cauſe or conſequences.

In this ſtate did Harvey find the doctrine concerning the motion of the blood; and although much remained to be done, as well in completing, as in demonſtrating the true ſyſtem, yet it cannot reaſonably be denied that much light had been thrown on the ſubject, and that ſeveral of its fundamental principles were unfolded. It would therefore ſeem that the writer of the elegant life of Harvey prefixed to the College edition of his works, was ſomewhat influenced by a partial attachment, when, after giving a judicious ſummary of the opinions of Servetus, Columbus, and Cæſalpinus, he ſays, "minime "veriſimile videtur, ex illorum igniculis "Harveium facem ſuam accendiſſe." We are perhaps wrong in expreſſing ſuch aſtoniſhment that the diſcovery of the circulation did not happen ſooner; and in placing it among thoſe inventions which may be at once ſtruck out by the genius and fortune of a ſingle perſon. A gradual progreſs may be traced through the whole: and it was not the diſcovery of any one organ, nor any one ſtep in reaſoning, but the concurrence of many anatomical diſcoveries, and many theoretical deductions, which was neceſſary for perfecting ſuch a ſyſtem. The Chineſe, who were acquainted with the uſe of the compaſs, the compoſition of gunpowder and porcelain, and the art of printing, long before the Europeans, are ſtill entirely ignorant of the circulation of the blood; as indeed they are of all the other important diſcoveries in anatomy; a ſcience which has never been the object of their experiments, and which cannot be much advanced by mere fertility of genius, or lucky accidents. With all the aſſiſtance Harvey could derive from his predeceſſors, there was ſtill ample room for the diſplay of his abilities: and he is fairly entitled to the higheſt honours exalted talents can claim; ſince that clear, compre-

comprehenſive, and penetrating genius, which from a chaos of confuſed facts and contradictory reaſonings, is able to educe a ſimple, connected, and demonſtrated ſyſtem, is certainly the moſt valuable and uncommon faculty of the mind. It is this preciſely in which conſiſts the merit of the immortal Newton, in thoſe of his productions which have excited the greateſt admiration.

THE method which Harvey purſues in his firſt celebrated treatiſe, entitled *Exercitatio Anatomica de Cordis & Sanguinis Motu*, is the moſt beautiful and ſatisfactory that can be imagined. After clearing the way by removing the errors of antiquity, he begins by deſcribing the motion of the heart as we ſee it in the breaſt of a living animal. Here he ſhews its muſcular nature, the alternate contractions of the auricles and ventricles, and the effect this muſt have, determined by the mechaniſm of the valves, in forcibly propelling the blood into the arteries. He then proves by calculation, that the blood flows faſter into the arteries than it can poſſibly be ſupplied by aliment imbibed by the veins;

 and

and as the arteries can receive blood from no other ſource than the veins, it muſt follow, either that the veins will ſoon be emptied, and the arteries more and more diſtended; or that by ſome ſecret paſſages and anaſtomoſes between the veins and arteries, the former receive again the blood which they furniſhed to the latter. He ſhews how this laſt ſuppoſition is verified in the paſſage of the blood through the lungs. Moreover, ſince by means of the arteries more blood is diſtributed through every part of the body than is neceſſary for its nutrition, what is ſuperabundant muſt go to prevent the inanition of the veins, as appears from their collapſing when the *aorta* is tied: on the other hand, the *vena cava* is ſurpriſingly diſtended when a ligature is paſſed round it at its junction with the right auricle.* Laſtly, from the ſtructure

* I CANNOT reſiſt the temptation of quoting ſome lines from a poem in the *Muſæ Anglicanæ*, entitled *Carmen de Sanguinis Circuitu a Gulielmo Harvæo Anglo primum invento*; and ſigned *Rob. Grovius, A.M. Cantab.* The experiment alluded to in the text is here deſcribed with all the graces of poetry, and yet with a clearneſs and

ſtructure of the valves of the veins, he makes it evident, that the courſe of the blood through them

and preciſion that could not be exceeded in proſe. Harvey is firſt repreſented as having laid open the thorax of a living dog.

Ast ipſum interea cupidum nova cura fatigat;
Quis cordis molem exagitet labor, unde calentes
Accipiat ſuccos, & quas extrudat in oras;
Quò fluat exundans per aperta foramina ſanguis,
Sanguis qui, inducto venarum tegmine clauſus,
Ambiguos trahit anfractus, & fallit eundo.
Sic ubi lentus Arar tacito per pinguia repit
Culta gradu, lenique pererrat paſcua rivo,
Incertum eſt partes has, an labatur in illas:
Cùm verò injectas accepit gurgite moles,
Et trabibus frænantur aquæ, vehementior exit,
Mutatuſque fremit, ſuperatoque aggere ſpumans
Sævit, & in Rhodanum violentas concitat undas.
Ergo placet tepidos amnes, curſumque ruentis
Sanguinis obſtruere, & nodo conſtringere venas.

Sunt geminæ ante alias inſignes mole, modoque;
Illam jure Cavam vocitat Romana juventus,
Hanc olim Graii dixerunt nomine Aortam:
Contiguis pariter labuntur fluctibus ambæ,
Et ſocios ambæ ſpargunt per corpora ramos.
Hanc Harvæus, & hanc oculiſque animoque remenſus,
Fortè Cavam primò tenui complexus habenâ,

them muſt be from the branches to the trunks, and not the contrary. This curious part of the animal mechaniſm, firſt diſcovered towards the beginning of the ſixteenth century by an anatomiſt little known, Johannes Baptiſta Cannanus, and after a ſuppoſed refutation, again demonſtrated, and more accurately deſcribed, by Fabricius ab Aquapendente, ſeems to lead ſo directly to aſcertaining the real motion of the blood, that it is ſurpriſing the conſequence was not at once perceived. Yet it was entirely overlooked by Fabricius himſelf;

Amplum intercludit filo cohibente canalem,
Obſepitque vias. Atque hìc, (mirabile viſu!)
Qui propior cordi ſanguis dilabitur ultrò
Cordis in auriculam, depletaque ſanguine vena
Concidit, & vacuas jungit ſine flumine ripas.
Qui verò excelſâ vitæ diſtabat ab arce
Longiùs, aſtricto præcluſus ſtamine, cœptum
Siſtit iter, magnoque attollit vaſa tumore:
Diſtentas tunicas, & clauſtra obſtantia pulſat,
Implicitos nequicquam ardens perrumpere nexus.
Poſtquam hæc Harvæus ſolerti mente notârat,
Ipſe manu nodos, & vincula linea ſolvit.
Tum ſubitò emiſſus per mota repagula ſanguis
In patulas cordis cellas, & tecta refertur.
Hæc ubi viſa ſeni, multúmque expenſa ſagaci,
Arripit ingentem, vinc'loque innectit, Aortam.

Omnia

ſelf; and does not conſtitute any part of the arguments of thoſe who made the neareſt approaches to the true ſyſtem. We are, however, informed by Boyle, that Harvey aſſured him he received the firſt glimpſe of the truth from contemplating the ſtructure of theſe valves, as exhibited by his tutor Fabricius; which circumſtance will give him a claim of more originality in the proſecution of his diſcovery, than he would otherwiſe ſeem entitled to.

THESE demonſtrative proofs of the circulatory motion of the blood, Harvey next

Omnia nunc diverſa videt, nunc altera ſurgit
Naturæ facies. Nam quà longiſſima vena
Perplexos ultra nodos porrecta jacebat,
Mollior elapſo flacceſcit ſanguine; ſed quà
Interius ſpectat, cordi conjuncta ſiniſtro,
Dura riget, ſuccoque ſuperveniente tumeſcit.
Allabenſque liquor, ſpatiis concluſus iniquis,
Æſtuat introrſum, vitalemque ampliat orbem,
Et propè diſrupti intendit retinacula cordis.
His etiam rite expenſis, ſimul omnia circùm
Laxat vinc'la ſenex; magno ſimul impete ſanguis
Emicat, & prono decurrit concitus amne:
Corque vices peragit, renovatque arteria pulſum,
Quantum efferre valent moribundi languida membra.

confirms

confirms by arguments deduced from the greater probability of ſuch a ſyſtem, and its perfect agreement with various phænomena both in the ſound and diſeaſed body. He concludes with ſome very curious and original obſervations concerning the differences in the ſtructure of the heart in different animals, and at different periods of life. He diſcuſſes the reaſons why in the cold animals, and thoſe in which the lungs are wanting, there is only one ventricle of the heart. All theſe varieties he proves to be deducible from, and accordant with the theory of circulation.

It was not to be expected, notwithſtanding the clearneſs and ſtrength of argument with which the doctrine of Harvey was ſupported, that mankind ſhould at once give up their antient errors, ſanctified by the authority of names to which the ſchools had been accuſtomed to pay implicit veneration. Two years after the publication of his book, Dr. James Primroſe, a Frenchman, of Scotch extraction, and an incorporated graduate of Oxford, publiſhed a treatiſe, in which, with a good deal of logical ſubtilty, he diſputed in favour of the antient doctrines. But his perfect ignorance of the mechanical laws of motion, and his servile adherence to Galen, whose decrees he argues from as so many postulata, rendered him an adversary whom Harvey justly thought unworthy of an answer.

Four years after, Æmylius Parisanus, a physician at Venice, published the second part of his *Exercitationes de Subtilitate*, in which he laboured with his utmost endeavours to overthrow Harvey's doctrine, and establish his own, compounded of antient errors and extravagancies of his own invention. This he attempted to do by authorities rather than arguments; and such, indeed, as frequently contradicted one another and himself. He was an adversary more difficult to answer than the former, on account of the strange obscurity and intricacy of his style, which rendered it scarcely possible to develope his meaning. However, Dr. Ent undertook the task, and with a mixture of argument and ridicule, exposed the weakness of all that was urged against the Harveian system.

A few

A few years after the publication of this reply, Joannes Riolanus the Younger, a celebrated physician and anatomist at Paris, presented his *Enchiridion Anatomicum* to Harvey, in which he had laid down a system of his own concerning the motion of the blood, in part agreeing with Harvey's, yet in other respects materially differing from it. He supposed the blood to circulate through the large vessels, namely, the *aorta* and *vena cava*; but by no means in those of the second and third regions, by which he understood the internal parts of the body and the muscles. In these he imagined all the blood was employed in the nutrition of the particles; and he supposed that the blood in the *vena portarum* and its mesenteric branches had an alternate undulatory motion. He likewise asserted that the blood entering the heart by the *vena cava* did not pass through the lungs, except in case of violent agitation from exercise or fever, but gradually transuded from the right to the left ventricle through certain pores in the *septum*.

Chimerical

CHIMERICAL and unſupported as theſe notions were, Harvey thought it due to the former reputation of Riolanus to anſwer him. Accordingly, he ſoon printed a ſhort epiſtle to him, conceived in the moſt reſpectful terms, in which, by arguments drawn from experiment, and from principles which his antagoniſt himſelf muſt admit, he refutes his objections, and ſhews the invalidity of his hypotheſes.

RIOLANUS replied in an epiſtle to Harvey, which contains little more than the opinions delivered in his *Enchiridion*, more diffuſely laid down, but ſtill unſupported by experiments. This gave occaſion to a ſecond epiſtle from Harvey, wherein he examines the nature of the blood in the arteries and veins; proves that no efferveſcence can take place by which its bulk will be augmented in the heart, and thus produce a diſtenſion of the heart and arteries; that the imaginary ſeparation of the vital ſpirits by means of the heart, cannot take place; and that the arteries are not to be conſidered as containing a flatulent humour of a peculiar nature,

but

but the blood by which every part of the body is nouriſhed and ſupported. He alſo, by proper experiments, demonſtrates the paſſage of the blood from the meſenteric arteries to the *vena portarum*, and the impoſſibility of a reflux of the blood from the veins to the arteries.

Riolanus, ſtill unwilling to yield, rejoined in a ſecond epiſtle, in which he expreſſes ſome doubts concerning Harvey's experiments; though, as appears, on no other foundation than that they diſagreed with his hypotheſes, and that he had not made any himſelf. Harvey, finding that arguments were of no avail in convincing his antagoniſt, dropt the debate. Some opponents ſtill remained; but Harvey, who in his diſpute with Riolanus, had anſwered all the moſt important objections which could be raiſed againſt his doctrine, did not think himſelf obliged to engage any further in the controverſy. Beſides, the truth now began to be ſupported by men of reputation in various parts of Europe; and Harvey had the uncommon felicity of ſeeing his diſcovery completely eſtabliſhed before his

his death. His treatiſes are ſtill conſidered, in point of clearneſs of method, and ſolidity of argument, as the capital performances on the ſubject. In two reſpects only his reaſoning is defective: his not attending to the contractile power of the arteries; and not admitting, or at leaſt obſcurely underſtanding the immediate communication of the minute arteries and veins. The former omiſſion muſt be attributed to the imperfection of all new diſcoveries: the latter proceeded in part from his unwillingneſs to receive any hypotheſis which was not confirmed by ocular demonſtration; and in part from his apprehenſions that it ſhould be miſapplied as an argument in favour of the poſſibility of a reflux from the veins to the arteries.

With regard to the invidious attempts to rob him of his due ſhare of honour, by induſtriouſly ſearching for proofs of the knowledge of the circulation, in the obſcure words and phraſes of authors, who either were no anatomiſts, or who have in the cleareſt manner profeſſed theories entirely different, they cannot, now prejudice and envy have ſubſided, require

require a refutation. It has, I imagine, been sufficiently shewn, that this important doctrine is not of a kind which could have been fallen upon casually and without premeditation: and where we are certain that the proper means could not have been used, we have sufficient reason to discredit the pretended effects.

Harvey's other great work, concerning *Generation*, as it consists chiefly of a detail of facts and observations, will not easily admit of an analysis. We shall however attempt to give a general idea of its nature, and the advances made in it towards the elucidation of this difficult subject.

It consists of sixty-two separate *exercitations*; and eight more, additional to the rest. The object is to detect the nature of conception, and the origin and progress of the new animal. He takes for his chief example the hen and chick, from the ease with which this species can be procured, and the certainty to be obtained respecting the time of impregnation or incubation. After an accurate description of the parts concerned in generation, he treats

treats of the formation and growth of the egg, and the feveral parts of which it is compofed. He then, from a daily infpection during the time of incubation, traces the firft appearance of the chick, and its gradual progrefs. He was the firft who difcovered its origin from the cicatricula of the *ovum*, and who perceived the *punctum faliens* to be the heart. He accurately difplays, as far as the eye could inform him, the fucceffive formation of the feveral parts; and herein corrects many antient errors. He maintains, that the formation of viviparous animals is not different from that of birds; which he confirms by the defcription of what occurred in the diffection of deer in the various ftages of pregnancy.

The fyftem of generation which he deduces from thefe obfervations, is very fingular. He fuppofes that the blood is the *primordium* of all animals, and even prior to the veffels; that the female gives the original material, and that the male renders it vital and animated. He denies any mixture of male and female femen in coition; and that the male femen ever penetrates to the *ovarium*, or even to the *uterus*; and imagines the *ovum* to become impregnated, not by seminal contact, but a sort of subtile contagion, as he expresses it, affecting the female rather than the *ovum*. He thinks it impossible that a material cause can occasion impregnation; but as the mind by its action produces thought or conception in the brain, so he supposes something analogous to reside in the womb, which he terms *phantasm*, by the virtue and energy of which the *ovum* is generated.

This theory, though supported by various metaphysical arguments, must appear as fanciful as any of those which he has endeavoured to overthrow; and it may seem extraordinary, that a person who professed so much to reason from experiment and ocular demonstration, should adopt an hypothesis from its nature utterly incapable of such proof. A philosopher of an inferior class may be allowed to shield his ignorance under plausible conjectures: from a Harvey we expect proof, or a fair confession that it is not to be had.

The

The anatomical obſervations of Harvey, however, as they were made with great attention and accuracy, are ſtill very valuable, and except in ſome inſtances, where the microſcope has enabled the enquirer to ſee more clearly, they are aſſented to by later writers. He moreover introduces many very curious remarks in his work, both philoſophical and practical, on matters connected with his principal ſubject. Such are thoſe on abortions; on tubal conceptions; on hermaphrodites; on difficult labours; and on various diſeaſes of the *uterus*. The obſervations on the generation of inſects, which were ſo unfortunately loſt, would, doubtleſs, have made a very valuable addition to this work.

A short piece, giving an account of the diſſection of Thomas Parr, who died in his hundred and fifty-third year; and ſome epiſtles to learned foreign phyſicians, extracted from the papers of Sir George Ent, are all the remains of this great man which have been publiſhed. The epiſtles were firſt printed in a ſplendid and accurate edition of his works, which the College of Phyſicians, much to their honour, preſented to the learned world in 1766, as the beſt monument of their illuſtrious colleague and benefactor. I have already mentioned the elegant Latin life of Harvey prefixed to this edition; to which I muſt acknowledge great obligations in the compilation of this article.

With reſpect to the ſtyle of Harvey's works, it is, perhaps, a circumſtance deſerving commendation, that, when treating on ſubjects ſo perfectly modern, he did not confine himſelf within the rules of ſtrict latinity, but uſed, without ſcruple, ſuch technical terms, as had been found neceſſary to expreſs the ideas of an improved ſcience. This is principally applicable to his treatiſes on the motion of the blood; in which, wholly intent on his ſubject, he appears only ſolicitous to write intelligibly, and inattentive to elegance. His book on generation is written in a language more pure and flowing; and from many paſſages in which the ſubject gives room for the diſplay of eloquence, it ſufficiently appears that he was no inconſiderable maſter of of fine writing, and capable of ſupporting that claſſical reputation, which has adorned the character of ſo many Engliſh phyſicians.

The following liſt is given of works which Harvey had planned or written, but were loſt in the plunder of his houſe during the civil wars.

A Practice of Phyſic, conformable to the Doctrine of the Circulation.

Obſervationes de Uſu Lienis.

Obſervationes de Motu Locali.

Tractatus de Pulmonum Uſu & Motu, &c.

Tractatus de Animalium Amore, Libidine & Coitu.

Obſervationes Medicinales. (Thoſe in the Britiſh Muſeum in Harvey's name appear not to be genuine.)

Anatomia Medica ad Medicinæ Uſum maxime accomodata.

De Nutritionis Modo.

FRANCIS GLISSON

WAS born at Rampisham in Dorsetshire in the year 1597, and educated in Caius college, Cambridge, of which he became fellow; and in 1627 was incorporated M. A. in Oxford. He then applied himself to the study of physic, in which faculty he took his degree of doctor at Cambridge; and in that university was made Regius Professor of physic, which office he held about forty years.*

HE settled in London for the practice of his profession; and was admitted a candidate of the College of Physicians in 1634, and fellow the year after. In 1639 he was chosen

* THE famous mathematician, Dr. Wallis, studying the speculative parts of medicine and anatomy at the university, kept his public exercise in those branches of science under Dr. Glisson; and was the first of the doctor's pupils who in a public disputation maintained the doctrine of the circulation.

Biogr. Brit. art. Wallis.

Anatomy

Anatomy Reader in the College; and in that department acquired great reputation by his lectures *De Morbis Partium*, which he was particularly requested by his colleagues to make public. During the civil wars he retired to Colchester, where he practised with great credit in those times of confusion; and was in the town at its memorable siege by the parliament forces in 1648.

He was one of that small but illustrious society, who, as we are informed by Dr. Wallis, one of the members, instituted a weekly meeting in London about the year 1645, for the purpose of promoting enquiries into natural and experimental philosophy. In the years 1648 and 49, several of the members removing to Oxford on account of the civil commotions, renewed their meeting in that city; while at the same time the members remaining at London assembled as before. After the Restoration, the meetings in London being augmented by the return and accession of several eminent persons, at length happily issued in the institution of the *Royal Society*;

 of

of which Dr. Gliſſon became, of courſe, a member.*

In 1650, he publiſhed his treatiſe *De Rachitide, ſeu Morbo Puerili*; and in 1654, that *De Hepate*. In 1655, he was created one of the elects of the College, of which learned body he afterwards was ſeveral years preſident. During the rage of the plague in 1665, he continued in London, and viſited many patients, but eſcaped the infection. The method he uſed for preſervation was thruſting bits of ſponge dipped in vinegar up his noſtrils. Sir Theodore Mayerne has mentioned, upon the authority of Dr. Bate, a remedy uſed by Gliſſon for himſelf in another caſe. He had been three weeks afflicted with a ſevere vertigo, when, after other remedies had failed, he was cured by a plaſter of flowers of ſulphur and white of egg applied to the whole head, cloſe ſhaven. †

* The beſt account of the origin and progreſs of theſe philoſophical meetings is to be met with in the preface to Dr. Ward's *Lives of Greſham Profeſſors*.

† *Prax. Mayern.* 44.

In

In 1672, Gliſſon printed his *Tractatus de Natura Subſtantiæ Energeticæ.* This work is dedicated to Anthony Aſhley, earl of Shafteſbury; and in the epiſtle dedicatory, he mentions having been for ſeveral years phyſician in ordinary to this nobleman and his family, and acknowledges the obligations he lay under to him for his patronage and aſſiſtance in ſeveral difficulties he had met with.

In 1677, he publiſhed his book *De Ventriculo & Inteſtinis*; and during the courſe of this year he died, in the pariſh of St. Bride's, London, aged eighty; leaving behind him the character of a very worthy, as well as a learned and able man.

He was one of the firſt of that group of Engliſh anatomiſts, who, incited by the great example of Harvey, purſued their enquiries into the human ſtructure, as it were in concert, and with more ardour and ſucceſs than their countrymen ever ſince that period have done. Of theſe, none exceeded Gliſſon in judgment and accuracy; inſomuch that Boerhaave terms him "omnium Anatomicorum "exactiſ-

"exactiſſimus;" and Haller, ſpeaking of one of his books, ſays, "Egregius liber, ut ſolent "hujus viri eſſe."

His firſt work, the *Treatiſe on the Rickets*, on ſeveral accounts deſerves particular notice. The preface mentions that five years* before the publication of this book, the following fellows of the College of Phyſicians, Drs. F. Gliſſon, T. Sheaf, G. Bate, A. Regemorter, J. Wright, N. Paget, J. Goddard, and E. French, members of a private ſociety for the improvement of their profeſſion, had communicated to each other written obſervations concerning this new diſeaſe. From theſe it was thought proper to make extracts, and to compoſe an expreſs treatiſe on the ſubject; the care of which was unanimouſly delegated to Drs. Gliſſon, Bate and Regemorter. The plan at firſt agreed on by theſe gentlemen was, that each ſhould take a ſeparate part of the work, and complete it. But on Dr. Gliſſon's

* It is to be obſerved, that Dr. Whiſtler had written a treatiſe on the rickets five years before this was publiſhed; ſo that this ſpecification of time is not without a particular purpoſe.

finiſhing

finifhing his, which contained an inveftigation of the caufe of the difeafe, to the fatiffaction of the other two, but with many opinions peculiar to himfelf, they changed their defign, and committed to him the planning of the whole work, that all its parts might be congruous and dependent on each other. This Gliffon accepted, on the condition that they would ftill affift him with their advice and judgment, and contribute their own obfervations. In this manner was the work compofed.

The *hiftory of the difeafe* informs us that it appeared, about thirty years before the writing of this treatife, in the counties of Dorfet and Somerfet. From hence it gradually fpread over all the fouthern and weftern parts of the kingdom, but was fcarcely then commonly known in the north. The vulgar name univerfally ufed for it was the rickets; yet on the clofeft enquiry, the author of this name could never be difcovered. Its affinity with the later invented fcientific Greek name *rachitis* was the caufe of much debate, fome fuppofing the unknown author of the name had, from obfervation observation of the affection of the ſpine, given it a denomination expreſſing that circumſtance by an Engliſh word derived from the ſame Greek root; others, with more probability, perhaps, that it was a merely caſual coincidence.

The treatiſe itſelf begins with an account of the appearances on opening the bodies of thoſe who died of this diſeaſe. It is therefore one of the firſt ſpecimens of that inveſtigation of diſeaſes by anatomy, which has ſince in many inſtances been purſued with great advantage; and certainly, as far as it can be purſued, lays the ſureſt foundation for reaſonings concerning their nature and method of cure.

The ſubſequent deductions, which are made with all the forms of ſcholaſtic method, are; "That the primary and radical eſſence of the diſeaſe conſiſts in a cold and moiſt diſtemperature, with a defect and torpor of the innate ſpirits in the conſtitution of the parts affected. That the parts primarily affected are, the ſpinal marrow after its exit from the ſkull;

ſkull; all the nerves proceeding from it; and all the membranes and fibres to which theſe nerves go. That the tone of the parts is too lax, ſoft and flaccid, and the irritability of the arteries defective." Under the enquiry, why England is more ſubject to this diſeaſe than other countries, and whether it be really vernacular here? it is obſerved, "that indeed the climate of England, by its cold and moiſt temperature, favours ſuch a diſeaſe; but that ſince other countries are at leaſt equally under the influence of this temperature, its peculiar frequency in England may more probably be aſcribed to temporary and occaſional cauſes, and that therefore the rickets are not properly vernacular in this country." This opinion has been confirmed by later experience, which has rendered obſolete the appellation of the *Engliſh diſeaſe*, by which the rickets were firſt diſtinguiſhed in foreign countries; and has ſhewn that other climates are at leaſt as much adapted to their production as that of this iſland.

The practice recommended in this treatiſe is judiciouſly accommodated to the theory of its

its nature and cauſe; and although overloaded with medicinal articles, many of them very compound, according to the faſhion of the times, yet may be conſidered as ſtill worthy of imitation. Rhubarb and ſteel are particularly recommended among the internal medicines; the latter, however, adminiſtered with particular caution. Exerciſe and friction are at the head of the external; but the cold bath was not yet adopted: on the contrary, a good degree of warmth in the liquors or unguents rubbed in, is approved.

It was tranſlated into Engliſh, the year after its publication, by Philip Armin, and alſo about the ſame time by Nicholas Culpepper. The original has been ſeveral times reprinted both in England and abroad.

His next work, entitled *Anatome Hepatis*, contains a much more exact deſcription of that *viſcus* than had before appeared. Though he by no means exhauſted the ſubject, having examined but few human livers, and thoſe out of the body, yet he traced many parts with more accuracy than his predeceſſors had done.

done. The capſule of the *vena portarum* has been ſuppoſed firſt diſcovered by him, and has ever ſince borne his name; yet Waleus and Pecquet had ſeen it ſomewhat before, and he has only the merit of having firſt examined and deſcribed it with accuracy; as he likewiſe did the branches of the *vena portarum*, its ſinus, and the bile veſſels; adding a juſt theory of the motion of the bile. He argues againſt the ſanguific power of the liver, and ſhews that the veins have not their origin from it. He ſubjoins many obſervations concerning the lymphatic veſſels, and on nutrition and ſecretion as proceeding from the nerves; together with conjectures on the uſe of the ſpleen, and other glands. This piece, which was ſeveral times reprinted, gained him the higheſt reputation in the anatomical world. It appears that he made uſe of anatomical injections, and he has given a figure of his tube for that purpoſe.

His laſt publication, the treatiſe *De Ventriculo & Inteſtinis*, contains every thing at that time known concerning the alimentary canal, diſpoſed in a clear method, with various

various new obſervations. In this work he gives the firſt idea of the nature of a ſimple fibre, and the irritable principle reſiding in the ſolids. He imputes the action of the heart to irritability, which he divides, according to its degree, into too great and too little, diſtinguiſhing it from ſenſation, and even firſt inventing its name. He has many remarks relative to muſcular motion; and mentions the celebrated experiment, by which it is proved that the bulk of a muſcle in action is diminiſhed, rather than increaſed. The invention of this experiment is, however, by ſome attributed, upon the authority of the regiſter of the Royal Society, to Dr. Goddard. He treats largely on the antiperiſtaltic motion of the inteſtines; and ſuppoſes, contrary to the common opinion at that time, that the inteſtines are not compoſed merely of membrane, but have a conſiderable quantity of glandulous *parenchyma*. He was almoſt the firſt after Fallopius who ſeparated the *palatum molle* from the *uvula*. Numerous obſervations, phyſiological and pathological, are interſperſed through the work; which, however,

ever, has, upon the whole, leſs anatomical merit than his deſcription of the liver.

DR. GLISSON's largeſt work is a metaphyſical piece, the title of which at length is

Tractatus de Natura Subſtantiæ Energetica, ſeu de Vita Naturæ, ejuſque tribus primis Facultatibus

Perceptiva
Appetitiva & } *Naturalibus.*
Motiva

IT is a moſt profound and laborious performance, in the very depths of the Ariſtotelic philoſophy, with all its numerous diviſions; and though in a ſyſtem and manner now out of vogue, deſerves admiration as an extraordinary effort of the underſtanding in a man of an advanced age. In it, he ſupports the opinion that the cauſe of motion reſides in the body itſelf, and does not ſubſiſt in animals alone.

THE reſt of the Engliſh Anatomiſts of the *Harveian School,* as Ent, Highmore, Jolliffe,

Scarborough, were born ſo much later, that they do not properly come within the period preſcribed to the *preſent part* of this work.

INDEX.

INDEX.

A.

INDEX.

B.

C.

Caſe

INDEX.

INDEX.

D.

Ebony

INDEX.

E.

F.

G.

INDEX.

H.

I.

K.

L.

Linacre,

INDEX.

Parifanus,

I N D E X.

P.

R.

S.

Scotch

Venner,

I N D E X.

T H E   E N D.

Printed in the United States
By Bookmasters